PINELAND'S PAST

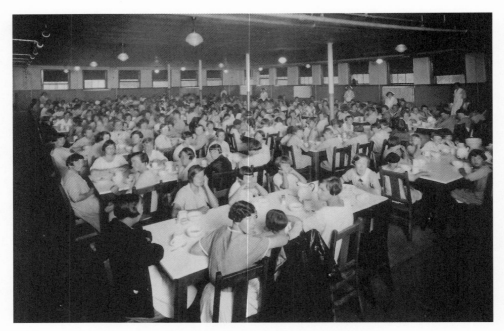

Girls at mealtime (courtesy of the New Gloucester Historical Society)

PINELAND'S PAST

The first one hundred years

by

Richard S. Kimball

Foreword by Governor Angus S. King, Jr.

Peter E. Randall Publisher
Portsmouth, New Hampshire
2001

Design: Grace Peirce

Library of Congress Cataloging-in-Publication Data

Pinelands past : the first one hundrd years / by Richard S. Kimball ; foreword by
Angus S. King, Jr.
          p. cm.
Includes index.
ISBN 0-914339-98-2 (alk. paper)
1. Pineland Center (New Gloucester, Me)--History. 2. Developmentally disabled
--Institutional care--Maine--Case studies. I. Title.
HV1570.5.U6 M225 2001
362.1'968--dc21

2001048224

Distributed by University Press of New England
          Hanover and London

Peter E. Randall Publisher
Box 4726, Portsmouth, NH 03802-4726

To the makers of Pineland's past
and the dreamers of Pineland's future

The fact that we are human beings is infinitely more important than all the peculiarities that distinguish human beings from one another.

—Simone de Beauvoir

Contents

Foreword by Gov. Angus S. King, Jr xi

Preface xiii

Credits xxi

List of Illustrations xxiii

Part One. Protecting People Outside by Putting People Inside
   1. Rocky Beginnings: 1903–1919 3
   2. The Vosburgh Years: 1919–1937 27
   3. The Kupelian Years: 1938–1953 53

Part Two. Protecting People Inside by Putting Them Outside
   4. The Bowman Years: 1953–1972 83
   5. Division and Consent: The 1970s 121
   6. Ascent and Decline: The 1980s 159
   7. Closure: 1990–1996 195

Part Three. Preparing for the Future
   8. Respite and Rebirth: 1996–2000 223

Afterword 235

"Those Who Knew" 240

Chronology 242

Index 245

About the Author 257

Foreword

Pineland's Past demands a large and caring audience. I recommend the book for every resident and friend of Maine who is ready to absorb and understand it. I add that each and every one of us should read it, because Pineland's Past is our story. It is by us all and about us all.

True, not all of us have to cope directly with mental retardation, and Pineland's purpose through most of the twentieth century was to house and sometimes serve people with developmental disabilities. And not all of us lived at Pineland, or had family members at Pineland, or worked at Pineland, or knew people who did. Not all of us have even seen or driven past Pineland. Its corner of New Gloucester is far from Fort Kent, far from Jackman and Machias, far from Kittery, far, in fact, for some people who live in Portland. But Pineland is part of each of us just the same.

All of us together create our state and its institutions. All of us at times need the services we build, for all of us require occasional help and care. All of us give, and all of us take. That's why all of us together must accept responsibility for first maintaining, then improving, and finally enriching each other's lives.

Unfortunately, we don't always do as well as we should. That's part of the message of Pineland's Past. Sometimes we leave the job to others, sometimes we get our priorities wrong, and sometimes we push our problems out of sight where we can forget them. We did all these things with Pineland a few decades ago. We saw retarded people as problems and we locked them away to protect the rest of us as we went on with life. Later, prompted and prodded by some of the most dedicated and caring among us, assisted by federal funds, pushed by federal courts, and encouraged by philosophic growth, we made improvements.

Today we have reached the point where society rightly insists that individuals with disabilities are not themselves problems but simply people *with* problems—just like all the rest of us. We have entered a time when we look past disabilities to identify strengths and contributions. We have begun at last to try and welcome all who commit no crime and do no harm to join us in community. That's one reason Pineland has closed its doors. Former residents moved elsewhere—to nursing homes, to sheltered workshops, to apartments, to places closer to family and friends, and closer to the rest of us.

I like to think of this change as good. I also like to think of it as partly my doing—not primarily in my position of governor or public servant, but in my role as a citizen who helps support positive change, as someone who grows with his time in this movement called progress.

But my pride bears a price. If I may claim a part in making a better world, I must also admit a part in accepting and maintaining the imperfect pieces, the ones that needed change and the ones that still do.

That's why *Pineland's Past* is important. It shows what we did together from 1908 to 1996, for eighty-eight years when we were sometimes close to our best and sometimes close to our worst. We need to know such things about our past if we would forge a better future from our present. We need to know what our taxes do and what they do not do. We need to know where our public officials succeed and where they fail. We need to know what kind of a world we are building and operating. We need to know what we are doing to and for each other, because we are also doing it to and for ourselves.

Read *Pineland's Past*. It is a sometimes wondrous tale with real heroes and villains, with tears and laughter and joy, with comedy and tragedy, and with conflict that never ever ends. *Pineland's Past* will fascinate you, but more than that, it may change your view and deepen your understanding of Maine and Maine institutions. So it did for mine.

Angus S. King, Jr.
Governor of Maine
January 2001

Preface

History is a child building a sandcastle by the sea, and that child is the whole majesty of human power in the world.

—Heraclitus

I became a resident of New Gloucester and a neighbor of Maine's Pineland Center just a few months before reading that the Libra Foundation intended to buy the forlorn campus that had once housed many of the state's developmentally disabled residents and convert it to new purposes.

I liked what I knew of the plan, and in January 2000 I wrote a brief note to Owen Wells, the president of Libra, offering my services as a freelance author and photographer. He called two days later. Could I take pictures of the thirty buildings on the campus, inside and out? Yes I could. How many pictures did he want?

"I don't know," he said. "But I think it's a lot."

He was right. Nine weeks later I delivered two large plastic files packed with 2,031 color photographs. Together they captured a cold, empty moment in Pineland's time, and cataloged the crumbling conditions being left behind by the state. With the files went a letter that mentioned my intensifying interest in the place.

Winter Visits

Making the pictures had been an oddly emotional experience. The campus was buried in ice and snow during much of the February and March when I worked. The huge, empty buildings of brick and cement were as cold as any I had ever been in. The weak winter sun, shining through sometimes cracked and broken glass, cast curling shadows on wall after wall of peeling paint and disappeared into dreary, dusty corners, some filled with piles of plaster from the ceilings and walls above. The word *bleak* kept coming to mind.

"I've been in there," said Ellie Fellers, who often reported on Pineland for the Lewiston papers. "I think the paint is peeling like skin." I shivered at the image. "I took photographs in those buildings too," she said on another occasion. "I went through the bathrooms with all the toilets together and the day rooms with the broken glass and torn curtains. I saw stuff that residents had left on the floors, and patient reports, and notes about cockroaches. I could almost hear laughter and screams. The buildings were empty but I felt like a peeping Tom." So did I.

In basements I dimly lit with a flashlight, I watched for the motion of rats and the reflection of treacherous ice patches growing under long, leaking pipes. The few buildings still heated at first gave welcome relief, but their temperatures were much too extreme for my winter clothing. When I stepped out from one into drifted snow, my sweat turned to ice on my neck. When I entered another, I encountered a state police officer responsible for a dog training effort located in one wing. "Don't go into the room with the sign that says 'Dogs in Training,'" she told me. "Not if you want all your limbs."

"I won't," I said, and I didn't.

Pineland was not a welcoming place. Yet I found something more than decay in its empty, crumbling rooms and halls. I found more than the windows with bars that spoke of confinement and punishment in the buildings that had housed the most difficult residents in the most difficult times, more than the dust of history done. I found a sense of life and even love that had warmed those buildings in the near century some of them had seen.

When I found that sense in physical form, I made photographs nobody had requested. There was a tiny, now moldy Santa Claus thrown onto the trash when a Christmas celebration had ended. There were collections of crutches and protective helmets in the laundry, pieces of wheelchairs in another room. There was a centerfold from a girlie magazine. There were discarded pictures of residents on the floor, and forgotten pictures of their families and friends on the walls. There were crumpled instructions about how to help Susan P. and Joey H. and Annie N. learn to walk or feed themselves or climb stairs. And there were messages on chalkboards and bulletin boards, some darkly humorous, some angry, some friendly, some sad. "Welcome to hell," said one. Countered another: "Good-by! You know we had some good times here."

It wasn't much that I found, but it echoed life's pulse and it proved how very much some people at Pineland had cared. Seeing it and touching it, I knew that pleasure had mixed with pain here, and laughter had mixed with tears. Slowly at first, faster as I moved from one building to the next, I was drawn into Pineland's past.

So when the next call came from Libra, I was ready. Would I write a book honoring Pineland's history? Yes, I said, I would.

Doubts

Later, I had doubts, many of them. I knew from years of news reports—some of which I had helped prepare while working for Portland's newspapers—that Pineland's past had at times, to be gentle about it, lacked glory. I remembered some colorful, even wrenching stories involving residents and staff at less than their best, and I found more as I began my new research.

There were high points in Pineland's past, of course. Some of its leaders and employees had won international respect and admiration. In fact, Pineland officials organized and helped direct the First International Conference on Mental Retardation, an event held in Portland in 1959. In the 1980s, the center became the first in the nation to meet new court-ordered standards of treatment and care.

But there were low points, too. Through decade after decade, many legislators in Augusta failed to understand the human and financial needs in the place they didn't visit not so many miles away. Some caretakers used forms of discipline and therapy that appear not just primitive but barbaric by the standards of today. Occasional employees betrayed their trust by mistreating their charges. And some patients displayed their need for treatment by escaping control and torching barns both on and off the grounds.

People who wrote about Pineland frequently made strong summary statements. An editorial writer in 1944 called it "the Compassionate Heart of Maine." In the 1960s and 1970s, other writers routinely called it a "snake pit." Which was it?

Families had strong feelings, too. Through the decades, Maine's newspapers published letters from parents, uncles, aunts, and siblings both commending and condemning Pineland for its treatment of children entrusted by desperate families to its care. Who was right?

Perhaps Pineland was all the simple summary terms that people threw at it. Perhaps it was none of them. But it was certainly a mix of bad and good, of failure and success. Could a book honestly honor Pineland's past, even if part of that past seemed less than honorable? I reflected on this question for some time. The answer finally appeared at my feet. It came to me in the form of a bronze plaque that the melting March snow revealed on a rock beside the skating pond near the main entrance to Pineland's campus. The plaque carries the dates 1908–1996 along with these words of dedication: "This is a memorial to all the people who were sheltered here. And to the devoted staff, family and friends who endeavored to make it a home for them."

There in those words, apart from dates of legislative acts and buildings, apart from administrative action or inaction, and apart from inadequate budgets, was the essence of Pineland's past. And there was the answer to my question: Yes, it is possible and right to honor Pineland's past, for that past belongs in significant part to good and caring people who did their best, the people of the plaque on the stone beside the pond. What was good at Pineland was sometimes very, very good. What was bad was sometimes appalling, but also often controlled by events and ideas beyond the place. Yes, we can and should honor Pineland's first century, even while looking honestly at it.

Pineland's Past

Organized chronologically, this book examines the events of Pineland's history in turn. But that past should also be considered in terms of the larger history that encompassed it. *Pineland's Past* is too slim a volume to consider national and international responses to mental retardation in any depth. Yet I should note that the center in its first century was very similar to many other institutions in other states. Pineland's patients, superintendents, families, friends, and critics, including the investigative reporters who from time to time revealed its problems, all had their counterparts elsewhere. Most of the methods, treatments, and philosophies found at Pineland were also found in other states and schools. The love and care at Pineland were common to many other institutions; so also, unfortunately, was its neglect by many outsiders.

That neglect is critical to understanding and appreciating Pineland's past. Far too often, many of us outside such institutions left their maintenance to those inside, while failing to offer any substantial support. James W. Trent, Jr., makes this point in his book *Inventing the Feeble Mind: A History of Mental Retardation in the United States*, published by the University of California Press in 1994. His introductory words focus on the photographic exposés of the Lincoln and Dixon state schools for the retarded of Illinois. Taken by Jack Dykinga, the pictures are strikingly similar to exposures made later in the same decade at Pineland. Viewers saw much in Dykinga's pictures, argues Trent. But

> *We did not see in his exposé pictures of officials of the Department of Mental Health, the governor, legislators, or ordinary citizens—the creators and sustainers of state schools like Lincoln and Dixon, and in a sense themselves casualties of the discourse and history that lie behind the gaze we give to mentally retarded people.*

The history of our social institutions is our own history. We who judge places such as Pineland also judge ourselves. However, the intent of this book is not to judge but rather to honor the past by telling Pineland's history, the story of a singular place and the countless individuals connected with it. The story is not mine; it belongs to those who lived it. So *Pineland's Past* speaks frequently through the voices of Pineland workers and residents. It also offers pieces of many newspaper reports describing events as they occurred. These published accounts are second-hand but vital. They helped both to capture Pineland's most exciting moments and to shape the public's view of the place. They helped to determine the future we now have reached.

Pieces of the Pineland tale spark sharp responses in the geographic area of the institution as this book is written, for many of Pineland's neighbors have their own, personal Pineland stories to tell. Ask around in the towns near Pineland. Ask people what they know and think of the center and many will respond. They worked there or they were patients there or they volunteered there, or they knew somebody else who was or did, and they know this or that about the place because they have seen or heard. Some express pride and pleasure at what they know; others do not. Many express passion about the fate and future of the place.

"You know," said a New Gloucester resident speaking of an attorney who had helped reveal Pineland's problems in the 1970s, "it's a wonder he didn't get run out of town. People wanted Pineland to stay open. They had jobs there, and friends there. They didn't want this guy coming in and trying to close the place."

The truth is that the force of new philosophies, federal laws, and court orders was already bearing down on Maine. Pineland would probably have closed its doors in any case. If not that person, then another would have brought the light of late-twentieth-century opinion and wisdom to shine upon the center. That light revealed institutions all around the nation that had seen their day, and displayed new ways of dealing with retardation, supposedly kinder ways and more successful ways requiring deinstitutionalization and community integration. The sweep of history was far too strong for anybody to preserve Pineland as it once had been.

But this does not deny the importance of individuals to the Pineland story. The people of the place were critical to it. They might have acted within the scope of historical trend and societal shift, but they brought their own personalities, their own energies, their own causes and wills to their institution. They shaped the Pineland presence. They earned their warm credit as the people on the plaque beside the pond.

Debits and Credits

"I'm looking forward to seeing your book," several people said as I wandered about collecting information. "So am I," I told them. Now, finally, here it is, complete—I am sure—with some errors of both omission and commission. These are all my responsibility, even those resulting from misunderstandings of news reporters or others who saw and lived the story. I wish I could go back in time to get everything right, but I can't. So I invite readers who find errors to tell me about them in a letter addressed to me at 225A Morse Road, New Gloucester, ME 04260. If I accumulate a file of such notes, I'll offer a copy to the New Gloucester Historical Society so that they can be available for others to read.

A century's history of any institution as complex as Pineland is bound to be a bit confusing at times, but Pineland's story includes some peculiarities of its own. The name of the institution kept changing, for one thing. So did the vocabulary used to describe its clientele and the nature of their disabilities. People entering Pineland in the 1920s and emerging in the 1990s went in as "inmates," passed their last years there as "residents," emerged as "clients," and spent time along the way as "patients." The same people might have been classified as "idiots," "morons," or "imbeciles" at the beginning, as "dependent," "trainable," or "educable" in the middle, and simply as "developmentally disabled" at the end.

Pineland also seemed to bounce around on the map. Its boundaries did change from time to time; the property shrank after farm operations ended in the 1970s and expanded again in the late 1990s. But Pineland's buildings were firmly rooted in the soil and never budged. Early reports accurately placed it in Gray, New Gloucester, North Yarmouth, and Pownal. Its second name, Pownal State School, seemed to place it in that town alone, though the name was based on the location of the closest post office. Today most people consider Pineland a part of New Gloucester, even though it extends into neighboring towns.

The spelling of words was another occasional challenge. For example, the term that this book uses as "feebleminded" appeared in several variations—as readers will see in the quoted material presented by this book.

Another confusing point for people unfamiliar with Pineland is the repeated reference to its clientele as "children," "boys and girls," and "kids"—a usage reflecting developmental levels rather than physical maturity. It can be disconcerting to hear a group of octogenarians described as "kids," but that continues to happen even today in talks with former staff members and residents.

Many people gave considerable time to helping me find my way through the confusion. I list some here and offer my thanks, even at the risk of unintentionally missing others: Eleanor Ames, Diane Atwood, Susan W. Austin, William David Barry, Louisa Lowe Bishop, Mickey Boutilier, Beverly Cadigan, Mark E. Capano, Darla Chafin, Elaine Walker Christensen, Joan Collins, Kevin W. Concannon, Mary Crichton, Pauline Gelinas Dubois, Ellie Fellers, Joseph M. Ferri, Cheryl E. Fortier, Elaine Gallant, Wayne Haskell, Norma Higgins, John Kerry, Anne Koch, Phillip N. Kupelian, Conrad J. Lausier, Jeffrey R. Lee, Carroll M. "Skip" Macgowan, Dr. H. Jay

Monroe, Dr. Agisilaos J. Pappanikou, Rose P. Ricker, Nancy L. Thomas, Mary Beth Tremblay, Betty True, Edward L. True, Beulah Vosburgh, Nancy L. Wilcox, Neville Woodruff, Betty Wurtz, Conrad R. Wurtz, and Charles O. Wyman.

Several organizations and their representatives were also helpful. The New Gloucester Historical Society was extremely generous with its resources and the time of three members: Betty and Ed True and Beverly Cadigan. The Maine State Archives was quick to answer questions and assist with research, and the Department of Mental Health, Mental Retardation and Substance Abuse Services, in the person of its commissioner, Lynn F. Duby, was prompt and positive in answering my request for access to restricted documents. Employees of the Maine Historical Society, the Portland Public Library, and the Maine State Library were all cordially responsive to my requests for help; I am awed by the patience of librarians in dealing with people like me who are challenged by microfilm readers.

The authors of several earlier Pineland studies deserve thanks: John L. Hoffman, Ph.D., a staff social research scientist who brought a forceful social science perspective to his "A Brief History of Pineland Center" in 1983; Perry A. Hood, who spent a year of his Syracuse University School of Journalism master's degree program at Pineland creating "Pineland's 60 Years," a fifty-four-page special 1968 edition of the *Pineland Observer*; Judith Kleinberg, who wrote "History of Pineland" to fulfill course requirements at Bowdoin College in 1974; and E. Sedgley, who wrote the five-page "Maine School for Feeble-Minded, Pownal State School" in 1955.

My wife, Tirrell H. Kimball, showed considerable patience, too, as I invited yet another Pineland person to visit and share memories with me, and as the time I devoted to this project expanded well beyond my original estimates. Tirrell understood before I did how much I was learning from and enjoying this job. "It's a growth experience," she told me one day when I was feeling threatened by the piles of Pineland material in my office.

For the project itself I owe thanks to the Libra Foundation and its president, Owen Wells, who commissioned it, and to Craig N. Denekas, an attorney representing that organization. I am grateful not just for the chance to write the book but also for the fact that both men stepped back and let me go my own way once our agreement was made. I have not been asked by Libra or its representatives to take a stand or speak in any way to advance its goals for the new Pineland.

I can only guess how many other people would have responded positively if I had asked for an interview, but I am sure they number in the hundreds if not thousands. To any who wish I had called, I can only extend a wistful apology and an invitation to come forward whenever you want. I could not call everyone, even those whom others recommended. There was only so much time. But if I missed your important story, then send it to me now, at the address mentioned above, and I will place it in a file for eventual delivery to the New Gloucester Historical Society.

Looking Ahead

Pineland's Past ends with the beginning of the twenty-first century, but the story of Pineland does not. It will continue, I can enthusiastically predict, for many decades to come. As it unfolds, it may well continue the spirit and the purpose of this book. There is no better way to honor the past than to build on its potential, and the new Pineland is intended to do that. It should house many workers, welcome many visitors, and serve many causes, including those of people with disabilities. The hammers and saws now heard on the campus and the yellow tape encircling it like a ribbon wrapping a gift signal not just physical renovation but the arrival of a new era, a new idea, a new promise. They sound the hope that Pineland can and will fulfill that new promise. May it be so.

Richard S. Kimball
January 2001

Credits

Excerpts from *Inventing the Feeble Mind: A History of Mental Retardation in the United States*, by James W. Trent, Jr. (University of California Press, 1994), are used by permission of the University of California Press.

Excerpts from the Lewiston newspapers, excepting materials placed in the public domain by the passage of time, are used by permission of the *Sun Journal.*

Excerpts from the Portland newspapers, excepting materials placed in the public domain by the passage of time, are used by permission of *Portland Press Herald/Maine Sunday Telegram.*

The excerpt from *The Courier Gazette* of Rockland is used by permission of *The Courier Gazette.*

Materials from the *Maine Times* are used by permission of the *Maine Times.*

Excerpts from *The Bath-Brunswick Times-Record* are used by permission of *The Bath-Brunswick Times-Record.*

Excerpts from Augusta's *Kennebec Journal* are used by permission of the *Kennebec Journal.*

Quotations of Charles O. Wyman in Chapter 2 are taken from the video *Charlie Wyman: Making the Best of It*, made in 1999 by a group of Bates College students working with Dana Rae Warren of Moody Mountain Films. The quotations are used by permission of Dana Rae Warren and Charles O. Wyman.

Photographs from the Maine State Archives are used by permission of the Maine State Archives.

Photographs from the New Gloucester Historical Society are used by permission of the New Gloucester Historical Society.

Photographs by Ellie Fellers are used by permission of Ellie Fellers.

Photographs by Elaine Gallant are used by permission of Elaine Gallant.

Photographs by the author are used by permission of Richard S. Kimball.

Notes

The Maine Paper quoted in Chapter 6 encouraged reproduction in context with prior permission of the editor. Author research has failed to reveal an organization or person who could provide such permission, and the author regrets being unable to make contact.

"Those Who Knew," the poem at the end of this book, is taken from the *Pineland Observer*, an institutional periodical that carries no copyright notice. The author regrets being unable to find and talk with the poem's creator, Julie Parsons. Any information about her would be appreciated, and should be sent to the author at 225A Morse Road, New Gloucester, ME 04260.

List of illustrations

Cover
  Pineland Center in the spring of 2000
Facing title page
  Girls at mealtime

Chapter 1
  Hill Farm and dormitory on an early postcard 2
  Christmas cantata performed in 1915 6
  Valley Farm on an early postcard 12
  Holstein herd on an early postcard 15
  Shailer House 20
  Potato field in 1914 24

Chapter 2
  Boys cutting ice, 1922 26
  Girls' home dayroom 29
  Boys in class 33
  Pownal Hall 36
  Central kitchen staff 40
  Yarmouth Hall 46
  Manual training class 50

Chapter 3
  Beds in New Gloucester Hall 52
  Superintendent's house 55
  Industrial training class 61
  Window view 66
  Aerial view of Pownal State School 70
  Boy Scouts on show 74
  Kupelian Hall 78

Chapter 4
  A patient at his studies 82
  The new Pineland name 89
  Children's dining room mural 93
  Antiquated equipment in Kupelian Hall 97
  A plan for Tall Pines 103

An early *Observer* 106

Walter Soucy, volunteer 107

Pineland's driver training vehicle 114

Chapter 5

Pineland Observer, May 1970 120

The Church World, 1972 126

Tall Pines Day Camp 132

Writing lesson 137

Cumberland Hall living room 142

Observation post for spotting wandering residents 146

A fund-raising sign on the campus 150

Pineland Observer, April 1972 156

Chapter 6

A report to the court 158

Sculpted ice chair 164

Inside the chapel 170

Chapel bell and steeple 174

Pineland angels 182

Pineland's cemetery 188

A Pineland pediatrics room 193

Chapter 7

Stone and plaque beside Witham Pond 194

Pineland Center's *Observer* 198

Rooms for rent at Pineland 203

Pigeons flying free at Pineland's closing 207

Frederick Giguere in his new room 211

The key to Pineland Center 214

Charles O. Wyman 218

Happy clients.. 219

Chapter 8

An invitation to the new Pineland........................ 222

Questor's Pineland offering.................................. 225

Interior of Yarmouth Hall, January 2000 230

Chapel coming down.. 233

Part One

Protecting People Outside
by Putting People Inside

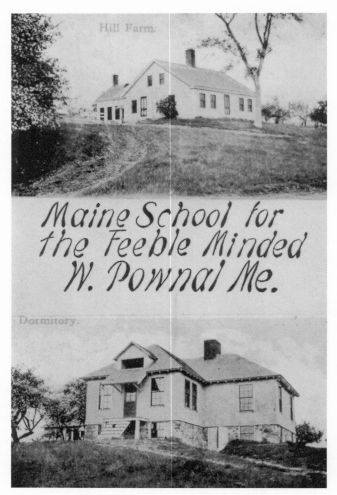

Hill Farm and dormitory on an early postcard (courtesy of the New Gloucester Historical Society)

Rocky Beginnings: 1903–1919   1

The past is necessarily inferior to the future. That is how we wish it to be.

— Tommaso Marinetti

Maine came late to America's attempt to build institutional homes for people with retardation. By 1890, the country had produced twenty-four such places, twenty of them operated by states and four of them private. But the Mainers then known by names such as "idiot" and "imbecile" and "feebleminded" were scattered wherever fate and accident had placed them.

Some were hidden at home by their embarrassed families, and a few were institutionalized in Massachusetts. Some were understood to live in "degenerate colonies" such as Malaga Island near Phippsburg. Uncounted numbers subsisted in town-run almshouses, which kept the poor who could not fend for themselves. Others, the "village idiots" of their day, were well-known and comfortably accepted by their neighbors. Many contributed what they could to the work of family farms and business enterprises.

But any general acceptance of the retarded was fast disappearing. As America became industrialized, individuals whose talents were primarily physical could contribute less and less. Fewer family members remained at home to care for those who could not survive independently. Reformers of the period and the leaders of the first schools for the feebleminded had begun linking idiocy with crime, delinquency, and lack of morality. Some also claimed that idiocy was hereditary. They argued, sometimes with fervor, that the feebleminded, if left on their own, would cause great harm by multiplying and producing more of their own.

The stage was set for change in Maine. Onto it, in the first years of the new century, stepped a troupe of reformers including Dr. Walter E. Fernald of Massachusetts, Senator Lindley M. Staples of Knox County, and assorted philanthropic ladies of Portland.

3

> The feebleminded are a parasitic predatory class, never capable of self-support or of managing their own affairs. They cause unutterable sorrow at home and are a menace and danger to the community. Feebleminded women are almost invariably immoral and if at large usually become carriers of venereal disease or give birth to children who are as defective as themselves. Every Feebleminded person, especially the high-grade imbecile, is a potential criminal needing only the proper environment and opportunity for the development and expression of his criminal tendencies.
>
> *—Dr. Walter E. Fernald*

A Call to Action

The ladies "made some startling and convincing statements" about the need for a new institution before a legislative hearing in 1903, said a news report of the time. Their voices were ineffective in that round, but the ladies continued their efforts the next year at the 31st National Conference of Charities and Correction held in Portland. There Dr. Fernald, superintendent of the Massachusetts School for the Feeble-Minded, described with great enthusiasm the progress made by boys at his institution. He even produced two boys for show, saying they had come from "isolated country almshouses," learned carpentry at his school, and emerged "fitted for a useful life."

Mrs. C. A. Weston shared statistics "showing the deplorable condition of the feeble minded she had found in making a canvass of Maine." To Mrs. Weston and to Mrs. Arabella Pollister of the Women's Council, said the paper, "credit should be given for doing the most valuable pioneer work towards arousing public sentiment in favor of the starting of a home for the unfortunate feeble minded of our State."

Among the aroused was Senator Staples. He used his strong influence in the legislature to win passage of a bill in 1907 dedicating $60,000 over two years to create "a home for the care and education of idiotic and feeble minded between the ages of three and 21"—later modified to six and forty for males and six and forty-five for females, except for state paupers, who could be admitted at a later age. Soon after its appointment by Governor William T. Cobb and his executive council, the school's first board of trustees hired Dr. George S. Bliss, a member of Fernald's staff, as superintendent. A committee led by the governor began the search for a location.

As the *Portland Evening Express* reported in 1909:

The plans called for a large tract of land, which should be removed from any large town or city, but at the same time easy of access by rail, on account of the large amount of freight which would be needed there. The committee finally decided upon a location which is situated in the towns of Pownal, New Gloucester, Gray, and North Yarmouth. The location is most excellent. It is but one mile from the Maine Central station in Gray, and a mile from the Grand Trunk station of Pownal, and is practically equally distant from Portland and Lewiston. It is on high ground and commands a magnificent view. Casco Bay is on the one side and the White Mountains on the other, being plainly visible, which means an overlook of wide range of country. It further means pure air and plenty of sunshine. The tract includes 1,500 acres of land. Part of this is good woodland and there are many fine springs of water on the premises. The open land is fair farming land and the hay cut is excellent.

The job of buying the land went to Charles L. Dow and Albert W. Larabee of West Pownal.

One of the half-dozen farmhouses on the land was made into a home for Superintendent Bliss, and work on other new and old buildings began. In September 1908, the first residents arrived at what was now called the Maine School for Feeble-Minded. By the following summer, the population had reached the school's capacity of fifty-seven, and Bliss was asking for $100,000 in new money for each of the next two years. That was a fine idea, said Staples, who told the Senate in part:

I can conceive of nothing that will do so much good to the State of Maine as this institution. Those who have visited the Waverley [Massachusetts] institution and seen how those little, unfortunate children who are brought there, under the discipline and tuition of their masters, could not but feel impressed with its importance, and the good that is being done, and the discipline they are receiving.

The state shall establish and maintain a school for the care and education of the idiotic and feeble-minded six years of age and upward, which shall be known as the Maine School for Feeble-Minded. All such feeble minded persons supported by towns in the state, who, in the judgment of the municipal officers of towns or state board of charities are capable of being benefitted by school instruction, shall be committed to this institution.

—Bill passed by the 73d Legislature of Maine on February 28, 1907

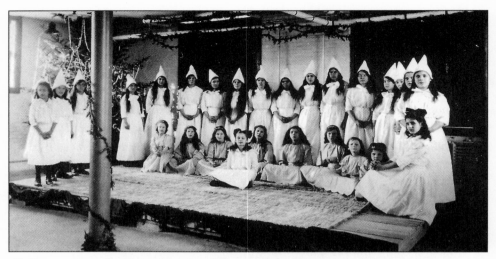

Christmas cantata performed in 1915 (courtesy of the New Gloucester Historical Society)

You know, as I said, that there are 2800 [such children] in the State of Maine today. It has cost the State year in and year out $27,000, from my investigation . . . for the support of the feeble minded by the different towns of the state.

Besides that we have been paying Massachusetts some $3000 every year.

If you give them the $100,000 asked for this year, and the $100,000 asked for next year we shall go home feeling that we have done a grand thing for the feeble minded and unfortunate of this class which we have among us.

Let us give it to them and stop the propagation of idiots in the different towns of the State. If you do, the people will not find fault with you for this appropriation, because it goes right home to the essence of economy and justice.

In 1908 the "Maine School for the Feebleminded" received the first patient to what is now known as "Hill Farm," after the farm had been purchased on authorization of the State Legislature. The legend has it that Dr. George Bliss, first Superintendent, arrived with horse and buggy and with the first patient who had been boarded by the State of Maine at the Walter E. Fernald State School at Waltham, Mass.

—*Dr. Peter W. Bowman, superintendent, October 1958*

The money was intended for a power plant, new buildings, sewers, supplies, salaries, and wages. When the bill passed, a period of rapid growth began. But it could not happen fast enough for some, who were busily compiling long lists of candidates for the school. In their early annual reports, the trustees and superintendents of the school regularly spoke in worrying tones about the number of applicants waiting for admission, and called for new buildings to accommodate them. The school's population was already 135, said the report for the year ending September 30, 1910, and two brick dormitories (later called Gray and Staples Halls) were nearing completion.

> [But] we now have on the waiting list over 300 applications. When the new buildings are all full there will still be over 200 left unprovided for. If we are to furnish adequate provisions for these poor unfortunates, we shall need at least $200,000.00 besides our running expenses for 1911 and 1912.

A Blissful Beginning

Growth came so fast that an early plan to adopt a "cottage system," housing small groups of inmates together, soon gave way to the reality of larger and larger dorms. Still, early news reports painted glowing pictures of the school. Excerpts from the *Lewiston Saturday Journal* of July 10, 1909, are typical:

> WEST POWNAL, Me., July 10 (Special)—The swaying of underbrush by the roadside and the chatter of boys' voices were the first evidence of actual work being done by inmates of the State's new Home for Feeble-Minded, as the Journal Wayfarer climbed the heights between Pownal and West Pownal, where 1300 acres are now devoted to the State's use. A few steps more and the group of boys could be seen working diligently with an attendant, hacking at the alders and willows and apparently rather enjoying themselves, if anything.

Farm products from the school for 1909 included 300 pounds of butter, 80 dozen eggs, 5 pigs, 2 tons of pumpkins, 16$\frac{1}{2}$ bushels of radishes, 177$\frac{1}{2}$ bushels of turnips, and 240$\frac{1}{2}$ cords of wood. Articles made by the girls in the sewing room included 16 dresses, 110 garter tips, 15 petticoats, 474 sheets, 42 suspenders, 534 towels, and 22 work aprons.

—*First Report of the Maine School for Feeble-Minded at West Pownal for the Years Ending September 30, 1919*

"Most people have no idea that we have inmates here as yet," remarked Dr. G. S. Bliss, Supt of the Home, who is by good right proud of the work already being done here on the hill. "But we have 11 girls and 41 boys to care for now and with our accommodations we consider this a good start. . . ."

Scanning the faces of the boys at their work, and later of the girls who were washing dishes, ironing, and helping in various household duties down at their comfortable quarters nearby, one noticed first of all that the children did not look vicious.

"These are not degenerates," commented Dr. Bliss. "I mean that they are more unfortunate than vicious. They are simple-minded, incapable of doing independent work in which initiative or any great skill is required. They are, as a rule, kindly in disposition, tractable, and obedient. We certainly have a good class of inmates so far and I believe this is the type which the State intends to reach thru this institution."

So far, educational work is relegated to the future, and it is only possible under present conditions, to keep the boys and girls busy and make them self-supporting as far as can be, while being properly cared for, well nourished, and made reasonably happy. By and by Dr. Bliss will be able to institute the classes in which an effort will be made to quicken these dim intellects and help to make these dependent individuals more independent. . . .

Among the "boys" and "girls," for that is the term used for all these inmates, were noted some who are over 30 years of age. The youngest is 10 years old. They are of New England country stock, for the most part, sturdy of body and possessed of rugged physical health.

"We have had little illness so far," remarked the superintendent, "and this is where Maine has a different class from that found in other states who draw their feeble-minded in no small degree from the large cities and the slum element."

The force of Dr. Bliss' comparison was more striking at the lunch hour, when the new and spick and span dining room at the Hill Farm was filled

---

I can't say I'm sorry to be through with the institution, for, as you can readily imagine, the associations there are anything but uplifting.
　　　　　　　—*Walter L. Kelsey, as he left his job at the school in 1912. He later returned and worked at the school for twenty more years.*

In the December issue of the Observer, there was the statement that when Pineland first began, in 1908, "Gray was about a one-day trip by horse and buggy from Portland."

We inquired about transportation in that era. Our kindly, learned, and encyclopedic informant was Mr. George Hill, a senior member of the Gray Historical Society, and a long-time resident of Gray. In Pineland's earliest days, the reported travel times from Gray to Portland were the following:

On foot - 4 hours.

Bicycle - 2 hours.

Horse and vehicle - 2 hours with an "average" horse, but 1-1/2 hours with a fast horse.

Combined transportation - Horse and vehicle to Yarmouth, and then electric (trolley) to Portland - 1-1/2 hours.

Train - From Gray Station to Union Station in Portland, about 50 minutes.

Automobile - ca. 1912 or earlier, about 45 minutes.

High-Speed interurban Trolley - This was installed in 1914 (and ran until 1932). It had a top speed of 60 m.p.h., and went from Gray to Portland, with stops, in about 35 minutes.

Perhaps the horse of our December issue needed a vitamin-and-iron supplement in his oats?

—John L. Hoffman, Ph.D., in the January 1971
edition of the Pineland Observer

with the boys at meal time. Their appearance indicated health and vigor of body, if not of intellect, and the appetite with which they made way with the wholesome viands left no room for doubt that few calls for medical advice are necessary here. . . .

But the work of the institution is yet only in embryo, so to speak. Dr. Bliss is looking ahead to the time when he can handle to good advantage 150 boys and 150 girls, if need be. Day by day the work is progressing to this end and the amount already accomplished augurs well for the rapid consummation of these plans. No time will be lost. Within a few weeks, in fact, construction work will be begun on one of the dormitories, probably by close proximity to the old Shailer place where the girls are at present housed.

"We plan to build two fire-proof brick dormitories, one for the boys and one for the girls, a laundry, probably of wood but possibly of brick; and a temporary central kitchen which will be of wood," said Dr. Bliss. "Later a permanent kitchen of brick will be necessary. Then these two dormitories will be augmented by the two colonies, one the Hill Colony now started on the old Lane farm, and the other the Valley Colony which is yet a plan for the future and which will be located at the old Dow farm now used as the dairy."

This dairy farm, by the way, is one of the prettiest on the State's land here. It lies in a fertile valley at the base of the hill and a mile away from where the other buildings are located. Here a herd of 18 Holsteins browse contentedly on the green slopes and furnish all the cream and milk needed for the employees and inmates of the Home. Here also are over a score of fat "porkers," young and old, which will furnish meat for the State's table throughout the year. Timber is plentiful over the 1300 acres and judicious and scientific cutting will enable Dr. Bliss to so manage that the two colonies may supply their own wood. Coal will be needed for the central plant later, of course. . . .

"Discipline?" repeated Dr. Bliss, when asked about this necessary adjunct to such institutions. "Why we need very little of it here. The boys and girls are good. Now and then it is necessary to send one early to bed or to deprive him or her temporarily of some amusement. This is all the discipline needed to secure obedience."

"What are their amusements?" was asked.

"At present we are proudest of our baseball team, on which there are two or three really good players. The boys like this, of course, and have enjoyed practice thoroughly the last few weeks. In winter there will be skating and sliding and by and by we shall have a gymnasium where systematic exercise may be taken, especially in the winter. Books, papers and magazines are read more or less and the graphophone is an unfailing source of pleasure to the inmates. They never tire of old selections no matter how often these are repeated for them. Then, too," added Dr. Bliss, "some of the inmates are musically inclined and we have several good instrumental players. Perhaps we shall have an orchestra or band organized at the Home in the not-distant future."

Some of the praise packed into the papers of the day went directly to Bliss and his wife, who was matron at the school. *The Oxford County Citizen* of June 3, 1909, had high accolades for the superintendent:

The feeble-minded may be roughly divided into three classes—the idiot, the low grade imbecile, and the high grade imbecile.

Of the real idiots there are only a few, nearly every case is susceptible of a certain degree of improvement. If a low grade child, who cannot eat except with the fingers, who soils day and night clothing, can be taught to acquire reasonably tidy habits, and to dress himself, the burden of his care is lessened immensely. . . .

While there is no sharply marked line between grades, the low grade imbecile is a better case for training than the idiot. In his case we expect to teach not only reasonable, tidy personal habits but also simple forms of work, so that the person himself shall actively assist in his own care.

The high grade imbecile is quite a different proposition. He is probably already tidy in his personal habits; he can be taught to read and write, perhaps to figure a little, he often has considerable musical ability, and can be taught to do many kinds of work well. His defect shows most in his relations with his fellow men. He is always improvident, always a liar, a petty thief, perhaps cruel to animals and children, and he may be so strongly inclined to setting fires that he finds the impulse impossible to resist. Because of his weak will and deficient judgment, he is easily influenced for evil, and is likely to become a drunkard, a vagrant, or, if a woman, a prostitute. . . .

Insanity is mental disease and is almost always acquired after puberty. Therefore, like almost all disease, it is a progressive thing and the patient gets better or worse, as he would from any disease. Feeble-mindedness is mental defect, a permanent thing that once established does not grow worse or better if left alone. . . .

[Proper care for all grades of feebleminded] is best accomplished by placing them in groups of not more than fifty or sixty in a building. It requires entire and absolute segregation of the boys and girls in their dormitories, in their work, and in their play. It requires sunny, well-ventilated, well-warmed buildings with abundant toilet facilities.

Until one has visited the school-rooms in a school for defectives, he cannot realize how difficult even such simple things as marching to time, winding thread on a spool, sawing off a board, or sewing carpet rags, are to some of these unfortunates. The effort that some of our poor boys put out, not merely to drive a nail but to hit it once on the head, must be seen to be appreciated. Many of the girls cannot do the simplest form of housework, such as to sweep and scrub a floor, make a bed, or wash dishes.

Most of them come to us entirely untrained, the low grade ones noisy and excitable or dull and apathetic. Many of them destroy clothing, will dig out and eat plaster, and break window glass or dishes. They can only be taught by slow and patient degrees not to do these things.

—*Dr. George Bliss, speech to the Literary Union of Androscoggin County in 1910*

The Citizen is pleased to say that Dr. Bliss, a native of New Hampshire, and formerly connected with the Home for the Feeble-minded in Waverley, Massachusetts, is without doubt the right man for the place. In these days, when officials seem to be tied down or held up by a lot of ceremonies and regulations, more or less indicating a dependence upon the latter, rather than an understanding of the spirit of things, it was a relief and a pleasure to find Dr. Bliss first a man and then an official. He is fully acquainted with the requirements of those committed to the institution and does not attempt to apply rules indiscriminately. He notes the needs of individual

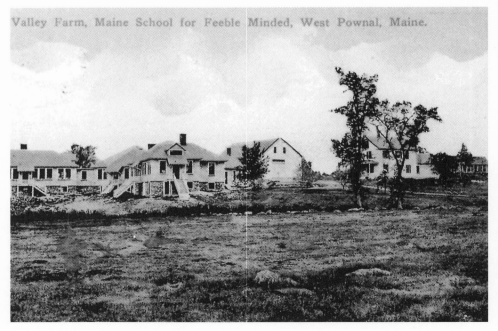

Valley Farm on an early postcard (courtesy of the New Gloucester Historical Society)

> The waters of Casco Bay glisten in the distance. . . . If these unfortunate inmates had a fine sense of beauty and an appreciation of the sublime they would certainly regard this as an ideal spot.
>
> —Lewiston Journal, *November 19, 1912*

cases. He was born and reared on a farm, and so is able to direct the farm as well as the educational work.

Added a Belfast paper of 1911:

We were glad to note that the Supt. and Mrs. Bliss as well as their corps of assistants, seemed to be blessed with just the right temperament to bring light and sunshine into their work.

Given such effusive reassurances about their new institution, Maine residents may well have been startled by the new headlines they read in 1912. Suddenly not much was right about the school in the minds of some legislators and reporters.

Squabbling Headlines

The reactions of readers must have depended in part on the newspapers they read. "MAINE HOME FOR FEEBLE MINDED IS INVESTIGATED," shouted the headlines of the *Waterville Sentinel* on January 30, 1912. "REPUBLICANS APPARENTLY OBTAINED FULL POLITICAL REWARD IN MANAGEMENT. Many Peculiar and Very Interesting Revelations Brought Out at Hearing in Augusta."

Months later, after committee investigations and probes and reports, the *Lewiston Journal* reaffirmed its support for the school, cramming much of its opinion into a series of extensive headlines above a long, illustrated article in a November edition of its magazine: "MAINE'S HOME FOR FEEBLE-MINDED Has Been Open Only Since 1908, But Is Prosperous and Fills a Long-Felt Need—

> A possession of push carts, such as Italians use for carting bananas, each hastened on its way by three boys or four girls . . . this pitiful procession came through the rain and snow and wind and sleet, bringing huge cans and tin boxes that contain food for 200 people. Thus, a small village is fed in this unsanitary unwieldy manner. . . . The state is not niggardly; it is lack of understanding more than lack of money that has left this condition so long.
>
> —Portland Express *report, 1909*

> When a legislative committee concerned about the school and its land made an investigatory visit in 1913, it "was served with an excellent dinner at the home and was informed that most of the food had been grown on the farm. The menu included fish and when some one asked what kind of fish they could get out there among the rocks Senator Packard promptly replied they were rock cod of course."
>
> —Waterville Sentinel

How Pownal Was Chosen for Location of Home—Dr. Bliss' Work With the Feeble-Minded—They Are Here Developed by School Manual Training and Out-Door Occupations."

The *Sentinel* was not convinced. "STATE MAY DROP ITS 'GOLD BRICK,'" said its headline on January 27, 1913. "THE HOME FOR FEEBLE MINDED MAY GO TO SOME OTHER LOCATION. Conditions at Pownal Are Said to Be Beyond Description With No Signs of Improvement."

What was wrong? Almost everything, according to the critics. The weekly operational cost of $5.18 per inmate was too high. The challenge of securing water from nearby rivers was too great. Construction bids for new buildings had not been solicited through newspaper ads. The population had too many "aged imbeciles" who could not be trained, and instruction was being ignored. The original purchase of land was suspect; it seemed that Charles Dow had negotiated for it without revealing to others that the state was the purchaser, and that some of the land was his own. The land itself was filled with rocks and so ill-suited for crops and animals that the farming could never pay for itself. Carrying food by pushcart to the girls' facilities from a kitchen 200 yards away was wasteful. Said the *Sentinel* after a committee of legislators had visited the home in January 1913: "Judging by the sentiment of the members when they returned from their visit to the home, if any town or city in the state has a good site for this institution, it had better get in its bid, for there will be a moving day in that vicinity before very long."

Not so fast, replied the school's defenders. All is well, and all can be explained. Dow did a good job and there was no time to run ads soliciting bids. The cost per inmate would decrease as the population increased, and additional funds could solve other problems such as the kitchen location. Some of the older inmates had been returned to their towns, making more education possible. Modern cultivation would improve both forest and farm.

So the debates went until early March 1913. Then the state decided to leave the school where it was—and to slash its appropriations for the next two years to

$175,000, less than half of what the trustees had asked. Water would be taken from Collier's Brook, a mile from the school.

The school was now under new management. In November of the previous year, Dr. Bliss had spied greener pastures and resigned to take similar work in Fort Wayne, Indiana. How much prompting his critics had given was unclear. In any case, Dr. Carl Hedin had been named the new superintendent at an annual salary of $2,000.

The Second Superintendent

Hedin arrived at the school from a position on the staff of the Augusta State Hospital. He brought with him full commitment to three ideas common to the times: Heredity is instrumental in producing feeblemindedness. The feebleminded are dangerous to others. And schools such as Maine's can and should train inmates but also keep most of those inmates permanently segregated from society. Said the doctor in the school's sixth annual report, dated October 1914:

> While it may be possible to support a certain class of the feeble-minded in the almshouses, we know only too well the disastrous result of such treatment of the feeble-minded as a class. The children receive no training, the men are often allowed to commit arson and other criminal acts, and the feeble-minded women are not given the proper moral protection which

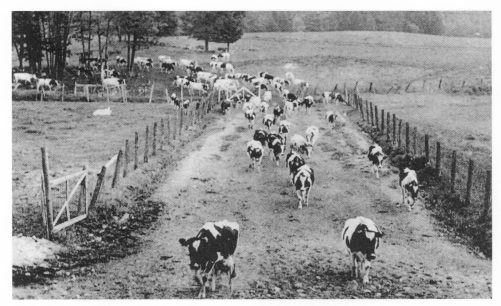

Holstein herd on an early postcard (courtesy of Elaine Gallant)

When I worked at Pineland there was the Nurses Home, Girls Home, Staples Hall, the old Shailer House, Hill Farm, Valley Farm and Morse House. The Girls House and Staples Hall accommodated seventy girls each in the two wards. Fifteen girls lived at the Morse House. The food for the houses was cooked in the central kitchen at the Shailer House—in what was formerly the stable—and wheeled in large cans and a cart over the boardwalk at each meal. I was an Attendant and then changed to being a Laundry Matron. I met my future husband at Pineland—he was an Attendant. When I left Pineland to get married I was earning $30 a month. That was in 1917. I have fond memories of Pineland but I expect it has changed a lot in the seventy years since I was there.

—*Alta (Haskell) Brockway to the* Pineland Observer *in 1987*

will prevent them from becoming mothers. We now know that morbid heredity is the strongest factor in producing feeble-mindedness, and we know that the feeble-minded are the most important factor in the production of crime, pauperism, immorality, and defective, illegitimate children. The public is paying for all this with ever increasing sums, and will continue to do so until the feeble-minded are properly segregated and prevented from producing their own kind. With this in mind, and knowing that there are several hundreds of the feeble-minded scattered over the State who are allowed to increase the public burden without restraint, there can be no logical argument against the crying need for enlargement of this institution. It costs money to properly segregate and care for the feeble-minded, but it will save money in the end.

The annual reports submitted by Hedin spoke of daily school exercises, though Hedin himself believed that the most important education came through giving inmates a chance "to do things with their hands." His reports also included tables showing the mental ages of new admissions as measured by the Binet-Simon Test, developed a few years before, along with the results of genealogical studies that demonstrated again the hereditary nature of feeblemindedness.

Newspaper accounts of Hedin's school had varied tones. Sometimes the reports stressed the negative, as did this 1914 article from the *Portland Evening Express*:

Even in the insane wards at Augusta there is no such pathetic sight as is presented to the view as one sees in this institution. Nearly 300 deformed, deficient and diseased inmates are housed in the various buildings and 175 are said to be on the waiting list. These inmates range in ages from small children to gray haired men and women. They are incurable and rarely is there a case where improvement can be brought about. From the very nature of their ailments, they are dependent and they will be wards of the State during life. Others will take their places when they die.

Sometimes the reports stressed the positive, as did this 1914 report on girls' activities from the *Lewiston Saturday Journal*:

A major portion of the mittens worn by the inmates are knit at the school. Many of the mufflers, which "bundle up" the boys thru the chill of winter, are made at the Home, and the neckties from the needles of the feeble-minded keep the boys and men supplied. The rugs are used in the various buildings.

Not many hose are knit by hand, but a knitting machine has lately been installed and, just as soon as the right kind of wool is secured, a pair of stockings will be turned out quicker than it takes to say Jack Robinson.

Because of the delicacy of the work and the care it requires, the lace making is, perhaps, the most remarkable feature of the industrial work. "Not many people with a normal brain would have the patience or the skill to do that," is the frequent comment of visitors, who marvel at the accuracy with which the girls handle the bobbins. The lace is used for trimming dresses, which are made at the Home.

Not only do the patients make these many useful things, but the older girls and some of the women assist with the mending. Dozens and dozens of stockings are darned by hand while as many more are mended by machine. Underwear is darned and patched. In fact, all sorts of repairing is done, and done neatly.

Aprons, shirts, and other things are also made by the inmates, under the direction of the seamstress. All of this work, in the industrial line, not only occupies the time and holds the attention of the patient, but aids materially in clothing the large family.

No insane or feeble-minded person or idiot is capable of contracting marriage. Such marriages are void.

—*1916 revision of the laws governing the school*

Whatever their individual reports might say, the newspapers of the time seemed to firmly agree with Hedin on the need for the feebleminded school. They also supported him personally, and the Lewiston article carefully stated that the super-intendent was quick to deal with occasional "inability or indifference" on the part of "undesirable attendants" who sometimes found their way onto the staff.

> *For instance, the story goes out that little or no attention is given to the teeth of the feeble-minded, that they are not properly bathed, that their hair needs more careful attention, that the cripples are abused by the other inmates, etc., and without stopping to realize that every story has two sides, many stand ready to condemn the institution on this evidence.*
>
> *No such treatment as this is sanctioned by Dr. Hedin. He is truly inter-ested in the unfortunates, who are placed in his care, and desires that they should have proper attention. He cannot be in a dozen and one places at once personally to supervise the daily routine, but just as soon as any such stories come to his ear he is ready to listen, immediately to investigate, and remedy the trouble if he finds it exists.*

The trustees, too, were pleased with the doctor. In their first annual report of his time in charge, they commended him "for his executive ability, tact and pro-motion of harmony," and for the reduction in cost of board by 50 cents a week, through "systematic arrangement of meals."

The Not So Feebleminded

One problem of the day escaped general notice: Not all the school's new inmates had feeble minds. Poverty, not retardation, was often the reason that peo-ple were sent to the Maine School for Feeble-Minded. Towns did not like paying to keep destitute orphans and others in their almshouses. They much preferred to

> Feeble-minded persons shall be admitted to the institution in the fol-lowing order: first, feeble-minded persons in public institutions supported entirely at pubic expense; second, feeble-minded persons in public institutions not supported as aforesaid; third, feeble-minded persons who are not in any institution of the state, who have no parents, kinsmen or guardian able to pro-vide for them, or who are committed by a judge of probate; fourth, those residing within the state whose parents, kinsmen or guardian bound by law to support such persons are able to pay; fifth, persons of other states whose parents, kinsmen or guardian are willing to pay.
>
> *—1916 revision of the laws governing the school*

> Whoever aids or abets any one committed to the Maine School for Feeble-Minded in escaping therefrom, or who knowingly harbors or conceals any one who has escaped from said School, shall be punished by fine … or by imprisonment in the county jail for not more than sixty days.
>
> —*1916 revision of the laws governing the school*

have the state pay the bill for care at the new school with the beautiful views. The state for its part was eager to squeeze as many bodies as it possibly could onto the grounds in return for payments from the inmate families who could afford it and for the physical labor of the inmates themselves—work that later critics would regard as "slave labor."

Getting somebody into the school was relatively easy. Town officials first had to apply to the trustees and secure a certificate from the superintendent saying that the applicant would be accepted. They then presented the document to the appropriate county judge of probate, who could commit the person once two physicians had certified that she or he was "a proper subject for the school for feeble-minded." In many communities, such agreement was quickly and simply obtained.

Transfer of patients back and forth between the state's insane hospitals and the school was also easily done; the trustees of the institutions could accomplish that with no court action at all. And inmates from the State School for Boys and the State School for Girls could be moved to the school with a statement from just one doctor that the subject was feebleminded. So youngsters sent to reform school for brief specific sentences sometimes landed for stays of indeterminate length in the school for feebleminded. They might even be there for life.

Looking back from the 1980s, John L. Hoffman, Ph.D., a social research scientist at Pineland, was aghast at what he saw. In the brief history of the school he wrote at that time, he said:

> *While employees could resign at will, the membership of the retarded residents was wholly involuntary. Discharge was possible, but hedged around with thorny restrictions, and relatively infrequent. Most residents quite seriously saw commitment to the school as tantamount to a life sentence. The school kept up a benign facade—sport activities, entertainments, and the festive observance of holidays—but any resident who tried to escape was usually soon captured and severely, even cruelly, disciplined.*
>
> *All too many who were not really retarded at all, and who could have functioned well in the community, were sent to the school as children, and*

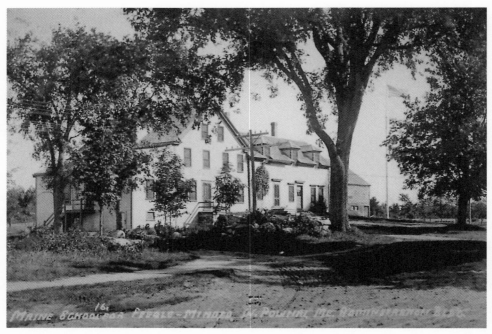

Shailer House, part of the school from the beginning until its destruction as a fire hazard in the 1950s (courtesy of the New Gloucester Historical Society)

kept there indefinitely. These came from low socio-economic backgrounds, often with broken homes, and they usually scored poorly on the early, academically oriented intelligence tests. In any case, they could be, and were, labeled as "morally" or "economically" feeble minded.

Charles O. Wyman was a case in point. He grew up in Troy, Maine, during much of Hedin's tenure. Disaster in the form of a house fire, a severe ice storm, and a debilitating flu struck the Wymans in 1918, leaving them so destitute that Troy officials intervened and placed the family in the town farm. Some of Charlie's siblings were sent to foster homes. But Charlie himself, though demonstrably intelligent and capable, landed at the Maine School for Feeble-Minded soon after the turn of the decade.

Malaga Island

Not long after taking his new position, Superintendent Hedin had to face the protest of a staff member over the presence of two residents at the institution, a mother and daughter from Malaga Island.

> It is hard to account for Malaga Island. Like Topsy, it "just growed!" . . .
> For a good many years this No Man's Land attracted scant attention. True
> it is that marriages were practically unknown. Men and women lived together
> and children grew up. Sometimes a Malagaite would trade his "woman" for
> a boat! Things became pretty badly mixed. White mothers—black fathers,
> and vice versa. Some children light—others dark. Deplorable indeed!
> —Portland Sunday Telegram *and* Sunday Press
> Herald, *March 27, 1927*

The state had wrestled with the question of what to do with Malaga since the 1890s, when newspapers began talking of "degenerate colonies" on coastal islands. Rumors flew wildly about Malaga. There was talk of inbreeding, strange racial mixes, idiocy, and poverty. There were tales that suggested incompetence at best. One told of a missionary who made a gift of shingles for use in home repair and returned later to learn they had been used as firewood. And it was known that men and women lived together without benefit of marriage. So troubled were the citizens of Phippsburg by what they had heard that they strenuously objected to the state's declaring the island a part of their town in 1903, and petitioned to have the act repealed. When they succeeded, Malaga—now called No Man's Land by some—went under state control.

When distressing stories and news accounts persisted, the state acted forcefully. In 1911, it plucked one family from the island and sent its members to the school for feebleminded. The following year, Governor Frederick Plaisted and his council evicted all forty-five remaining residents from the island, sending a few more to the school and the rest off to cope as best they could. That was not very well, because the surrounding towns refused to grant them pauper status and assist them. Then the state dug up the remains of the Malagaites' dead, placed them in five large caskets, and reburied them in the school's cemetery.

The presence of the mother and daughter at the school distressed a kitchen worker. Insisting that they were competent to live on their own, the spirited employee took the case well beyond the school, to the governor's council, newspapers, and elsewhere. But her campaign failed, to the condescending relief of the *Lewiston Saturday Journal*:

> *Her claim is that this mother and daughter are normal and should be
> given their liberty. She sincerely believes that they both would be compe-
> tent help and could easily be self-supporting. Dr. Hedin and the State offi-
> cials to whom she has told her story have listened courteously.*

> For whatever reason, no one has since come to live on Malaga. The arbitrary eviction of its population and the dismantling of their homes makes a shameful footnote in Maine history. No one would contend that the island was an Eden, but neither was it the iniquitous place dreamed up in certain press accounts. It was simply a tiny impoverished offshore settlement where people lived as best they could.
>
> —*William David Barry, in* Down East: The Magazine of Maine, *November 1980*

In the first place, considering there are one hundred and sixty feeble-minded on the waiting list, it can readily be realized that, if the authorities deemed it wise, they would be only too glad to discharge these two for the sake of others, who are desperately in need of care.

The superintendent and others have attempted to explain why it would be altogether unsafe to allow them to leave. At West Pownal, under supervision and where they have no responsibility, they are apparently normal but left to their own devices, there is reason to believe they would be harmful to society. Those who know the ins and outs of the situation say they do not doubt the wisdom of the State authorities, in keeping them under surveillance.

In this small story of the Malagaites are several themes critical to the larger story of the Maine School for Feeble-Minded: the power of the early superintendents, the difficulty of leaving the school compared to the easy act of entering, and the wonderfully supportive relationships that sometimes formed between individual staff members and inmates—relationships that would be seen many thousands of times in the decades to come.

The War Years

The First World War pulled some public attention away from the Maine School for Feeble-Minded. It also slowed expansion of the physical plant, but it didn't stop growth entirely. After all, the waiting lists were still expanding precipitously. New barns and other buildings appeared in the second half of the decade. A nurses' home, to be known as Sebago House, opened in 1915, and a central kitchen and bakery in 1917. The boys' building, later called New Gloucester Hall, was completed in 1919.

In a war economy, Dr. Hedin remarked in his report for the year ending June 30, 1918, "It is sometimes difficult to decide what improvements and additions should be recommended, and what should wait until a more opportune time." But he still came up with a list of immediate needs, including an electrical generator, a powerhouse to replace the shed that had twice caught fire the previous year, a horse barn, extension of electric lines to the farm colonies, and a woodworking machine.

The war years also brought pressure to increase farm production across the land, and the school responded to its best ability, said Hedin's 1918 report:

> *In response to the call of the Nation to "raise more crops" we have endeavored to raise as many vegetables as possible, both by increasing the acreage under cultivation and by improving several fields by clearing them of rocks and boulders. Unfortunately, the 1917 season was not very favorable on account of the cold and wet spring, followed by early and severe frost in the fall. The great shortage of employees, and especially of farm labor, also interfered, as never before, with the successful handling of large crops; and, therefore, some of our crops necessarily suffered materially from these causes. But in spite of these unavoidable difficulties, the farm operations were attended with fair success, and we realized a considerable increase in the production of many vegetables and other farm products . . . Much of this success was due to the faithful and energetic management of*

. . . I had a fine time driving down to the institution with an old yankee who found out what I was and how much money I had in the bank. I can not tell you what a good time I had up there. I enjoyed every minute of it. As it is I regret that I did not go up earlier in the morning and take still more of the New England atmosphere.

I told Miss Perkins, my matron, when I arrived home that it always seemed to me that when I went to other institutions they were doing things better than we are here. You certainly have a fine place started. Your farm is going to be one of the best, I hope. Your dormitories you will appreciate when you know that mine are so closely following the lines you have lain out. The splendid spirit about the place was evidenced in every corner. The fact is that I congratulate you and Mrs. Bliss upon the reputation you are sure to make.

—*Letter of July 30, 1912, from Charles S. Little, superintendent of Letchworth Village in New York State, after a visit to Bliss and the Maine School for Feeble-Minded*

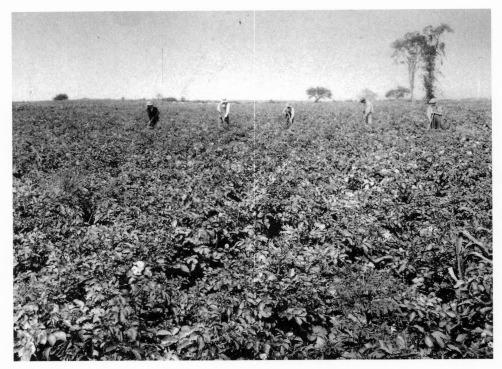

Potato field in 1914 (courtesy of the New Gloucester Historical Society)

the farm by Mr. Bartlett, the head farmer, as well as the willing assistance of all the boys and girls who were able to assist with the work on the farm and in the garden.

With the end of the war came many changes. The era of the prosperous American twenties was about to begin. Those alarmed by feeblemindedness would soon be wrestling with questions of eugenics and sterilization. And the strongest voice at the Maine School for Feeble-Minded would belong to a man committed to controlling the hereditary causes that he thought produced the school's population. He was Dr. Stephen E. Vosburgh, who replaced Hedin as the school's superintendent in 1919. Vosburgh came from the Augusta State Hospital staff, as had Hedin, who now became superintendent of the Bangor State Hospital.

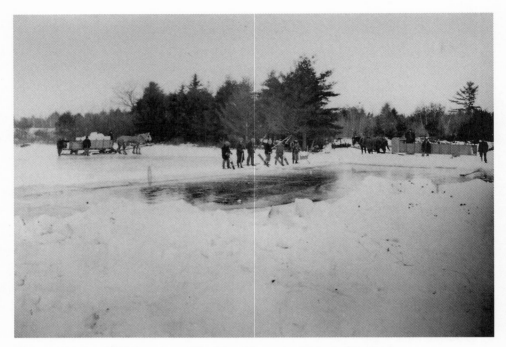

Boys cutting ice, 1922 (courtesy of the New Gloucester Historical Society)

The Vosburgh Years: 1919–1937 $\boxed{2}$

An institution is the lengthened shadow of one man.
—Ralph Waldo Emerson

An unlikely scorecard greeted readers of the *Lewiston Journal Magazine* Section on December 6, 1930: "In 11 years, a gain of 470 and 500 to go." This explanation followed:

> *Football yards? No. Beds.*
> *For those figures illustrate, in a word, what Dr. Stephen Vosburgh has accomplished since he took the reins at the State school at Pownal, and the goal to which he aspires for this useful Maine institution, which cares for the feeble-minded.*

Vosburgh had seven years of his superintendency still to go in 1930, but already the main theme of his tenure was clear, and that was expansion. The physical plant grew in the 1920s and 1930s, the staff grew, and the resident population grew. Even the expansion goal grew. When the *Journal* article appeared, the school had 700 beds and its goal was 1,200. By 1937, with more than 1,100 beds in place, the goal had jumped to 1,500.

A few troubling headlines had appeared during his superintendency, but Vosburgh enjoyed wide support, as the *Journal* article indicated with this fulsome passage:

> *Dr. Vosburgh is in the prime of life, giving the best to Maine in this capacity, carrying a load of administrative detail that would make a less mentally and physically robust man quail and quit. But he wears his obligations easily, has a poise that is unhurried and unflurried, is genial and kindly, not only in his relations with State officials and other outsiders, but with the children. They respect him, but have no fear when he approaches.*

The positions of employees in this School are sacred. They are to improve and cheer the most helpless of unfortunate children. To do their work properly they must themselves learn the lessons they endeavor to teach. To teach children to be neat and orderly, they must be so themselves. To teach children to be kind, obliging, and respectful, they must be so to each other. To correct evil habits of speaking or acting, they must be cautious of their own acts and words. Their chief work is that work of the School—to make the children self-dependent and useful in every way possible. Our motto is: The true education and training of girls and boys of backward or feeble minds is to teach them what they ought to know and can make use of when they become women and men in years.

Personal cleanliness, neatness in dress, and good table manners are required from all. Men are not allowed to come to the table in shirt sleeves, with sweaters, frocks, or overalls. If you are wearing a shirt without a collar, please put on a collar and necktie before you sit down at the table. A tie should be worn with a soft shirt with a collar. At the table, the conversation should be discreet and free from anything that might offend. . . .

Employees must not write to the parents or friends of the inmates without submitting such communications to the Superintendent for his approval.

The matrons and all others in charge of the inmates are distinctly and positively enjoined not to allow any female inmate to be left alone in any place where it would be possible for her to be alone with any male person.

While the inmates should be taught and encouraged to work, the attendants must not forget that they are employed to assume the responsibilities and work with the inmates. You are not allowed to stand or sit idly watching the inmates working, but must always work with them in every line of work. Do not treat the children as servants, but take the brunt of the work yourselves and treat them as voluntary assistants. Words of praise and encouragement help the boys and girls to do their best, while scolding or nagging discourages them.

—Rules and regulations of the Pownal State School at Pownal, Maine, approved by the Board of Hospital Trustees, October 15, 1929

*Here and there one will call him by name with a smile of welcome as he
goes about the grounds or through the buildings. A day's visit about the
place revealed this habit as spontaneous. For nobody could coach that
motley assemblage of sub-normal children into the numerous little acts
that directly or indirectly told this story to the observer.*

Such enthusiasm for the man and his opinions surely helped fuel his efforts
to keep building, even as economic depression descended and another world war
threatened.

Rationale for Growth

Why should the school keep expanding? Vosburgh and his aides repeated the
alarms sounded earlier by Superintendent Hedin: The feebleminded endangered
themselves and society. They should be confined for the sake of all. And the state's
problem was very large; statistical studies showed there could be 23,000 "subnormals" in Maine, Vosburgh told a Bar Harbor meeting of the Maine Medical
Association in 1925.

Therefore, the argument went, the school should expand until all persons sent
by towns and courts and families could be accommodated and waiting lists disappeared. In 1925, with weekly per capita costs at $5.75, the school had an annual
budget of $540,000 and assets valued at $1,135,000. But this was not enough and
growth would continue, Governor Percival Baxter assured a Portland audience on

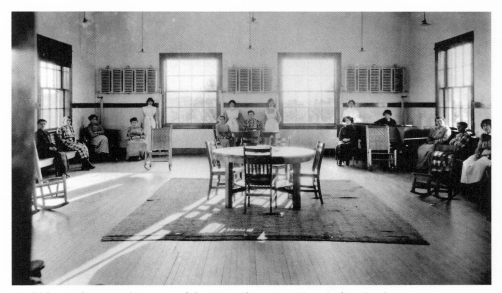

Girls' home dayroom (courtesy of the New Gloucester Historical Society)

May 15: "It is the fixed policy of the State to build additional dormitories at that institution until all the unfortunate defectives of this class are segregated and under the care of the State."

A newspaper reporting the speech offered full support:

> *Before the State undertook the care of its feeble minded, as it is doing to a limited extent at Pownal, these unfortunates were running loose in almost every community, defiling the morals of each, reproducing their kind, and adding to the pauper element of the population.*
>
> *Generation after generation of morons were growing up without let or hindrance, until in some localities there were whole communities of them, to add enormously to the burdens of the municipalities where they were found. From them a large proportion of the State's criminal classes were recruited and from them were drawn most of the inmates of the town and city.*

Vosburgh appeared frequently before civic groups. In a visit to the Woodfords Club in Portland on January 22, 1928, he described the education, farmwork, and social activities of the 750 inmates then present at the school. Formal training, he said, included school classes and manual, industrial and physical arts. Informal training included cooking, sewing, housekeeping, farming, electrical wiring, and other such labor that helped run the school and prepare residents for possible return to their communities.

Vosburgh also summarized contemporary approaches to treatment:

> *Three methods are employed for the treatment of the feeble minded. Good hygiene, which seeks to improve conditions before birth and in early childhood; segregation; and sterilization are the methods used, the most satisfactory results being obtained through a combination of all three of these methods.*

There is an amazing lack of correct information regarding the subnormal. Occasionally a well-disposed philanthropist believes certain subnormals of pleasing appearance who seem not too dull should never be sent to an institution. In general, the higher types of feeble-minded, such as the morons, are the most dangerous to the community and posterity.

—*Dr. Stephen E. Vosburgh to the Maine Medical Association, 1925*

Chewing tobacco shall be issued only to mature boys accustomed to the habit. Young boys are not to be encouraged or permitted to have tobacco, and no boy shall have an issue until approved by the attending physician. The use of tobacco is primarily to encourage workers and especially those who do continuous hard work. Inside workers should have a limited supply issued, and this is to be discontinued to any boy who is careless in its use, who gives it to smaller boys, or barters with other boys with tobacco as a medium. When boys are in correction, there shall be no issue of tobacco to them.

—*Dr. Stephen E. Vosburgh, notice to staff, 1932*

Hygiene was not frequently discussed in the news accounts of the Vosburgh years. But segregation and sterilization were, and dramatic news accounts of criminal acts committed by the feebleminded sometimes underscored the urgency of removing them from the community.

Fire!

The school enjoyed a period of relative calm during Vosburgh's first two years in office. But on August 4, 1921, readers of the *Portland Daily Press* woke to huge headlines shouting that "ESCAPED INMATE HOME FOR FEEBLE-MINDED BURNS 2 BARNS, CAMP NEAR NO. YARMOUTH." A deaf mute from Pineland had been found at one of the fires, the paper said.

When I went there Dr. Hawkes was superintendent down there. He was kind of a harsh man, I guess. We didn't see too much of him, really. Of course he had orders to give to somebody and they carried them out. But I never had any dealings with him myself, so as far as I was concerned he was very nice to me. But to some of the others he was pretty harsh.

—*Statement from "Henry Taylor," the pseudonymous name of a resident who entered Pownal in 1925 at the age of eleven and left in 1953. His interview was part of a study conducted by John L. Hoffman, Ph.D. The superintendent's name is also disguised in this report, but the dates suggest that the resident was referring to Vosburgh.*

The man wouldn't or couldn't talk but, when he was asked if he had set the first he nodded his head and grinned with delight. The men about him asked him how he had started the fires and the man made the motions of striking a match, touching the flame to something on the ground and then made a whistling noise with his breath to show how the flames had shot upward.

The people who were attracted by these fires came to the conclusion that they had captured the incendiary and some of them telephoned the Home for Feeble Minded at Pownal to learn the man's name. The superintendent there refused to give them any information and at first said that none of the inmates of the home were missing. Later he said that one man named Pleury had gone away from what is called the Valley Farm, about half past four o'clock. . . .

There was great excitement in the vicinity of the fires for a little while and some wild rumors were in circulation, one of them being that the incendiary had murdered a man named Brown who had tried to catch him in the woods. There was no truth in this yarn nor in any of the others which were stated about the desperate fight which the man who was captured put up. Pleury, if that is his name, isn't a desperate character, but is mentally incompetent and there seems to be little doubt about his being the cause of these fires.

Vosburgh's reports to his board about the incident had a calmer, more questioning tone based on the results of his own investigations. "It is to be regretted that this boy was away from the School at this particular time," he said, "as I still doubt his being responsible for the fires, it having been necessary to have covered four or five miles in fifteen minutes to have reached the first place." Pleury had no matches on him, Vosburgh noted, and it was possible that he had been drawn to the fires by the smoke they produced.

More local fires followed soon after these, while Pleury was safely on school grounds. In October a Gray woman voluntarily entered the state mental hospital

I wish to report that from our pasture one of the oxen became wild, broke through a fence, and is still at large after two days. We have several times gotten near him, but have been unable to capture him, up till the present. We are continuing efforts.

—*Dr. Stephen E. Vosburgh to the commissioner of Health and Welfare, 1932*

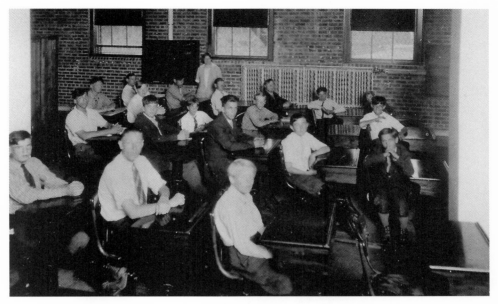

Boys in class; the blond in front is Charles O. Wyman (courtesy of the New Gloucester Historical Society)

in Augusta after it appeared that she had set her own family barn afire. Vosburgh passed the news on to his board, saying it was important only because "it relieves the Maine School for Feeble-Minded from further unfounded rumors that some-one had escaped" and was responsible for this latest blaze.

But the news did not prove Pleury innocent, either, and the link between fire and feeblemindedness was now firmly in the public mind. It would be confirmed for many in 1933, when an eleven-year-old Auburn boy was accused of setting some serious fires near his home. The boy soon confessed, saying he had wanted

My husband's boyhood was a strange one, living on the institution grounds. However, he learned much from the various projects going on there—farming, dairy work, etc. . . . My husband had many memories of the progress made there as he saw many changes as he grew up. He was also intrigued with the government officials and political visitors hosted by the State for meetings in his home. At fourteen he made a business of selling candy to the patients and employees.

—*Beulah M. Vosburgh, widowed daughter-in-law of
Dr. Stephen E. Vosburgh, in August 2000*

to see the fire trucks go by, and within two weeks he had been examined by the superintendent, declared a low-grade moron in the feebleminded group, and committed to the school with the consent of his parents.

Some experts at the time did express doubts about the connection between mental incompetence and crime. "The influence of feeble-mindedness upon crime has been greatly exaggerated," declared Tufts professor Dr. Abraham Myerson at an Augusta conference in 1930. "Our prisons contain many feeble-minded merely because the feeble-minded are easily caught. The mere possession of a mind somewhat below normal does not necessarily mean that its possessor will become a criminal." But Myerson's was a minority view. For years to come, Maine would remain committed to removing the feebleminded from society. Moreover, it was already taking firm steps to prevent their reproduction.

Sterilization

By the middle of the 1920s, some experts on feeblemindedness were beginning to point out that its causes were often not hereditary. One was Dr. Walter E. Fernald, whose work at the Massachusetts School for the Feeble-Minded had helped prepare the way for the Maine institution. But Vosburgh and others in Maine firmly disagreed. Among the superintendent's most vociferous supporters were Judge Lauren M. Sanborn, of Cumberland County Superior Court, who apparently spoke out of his experience dealing with criminals in his courtroom, and Senator Alexander Spiers of Cumberland County. Spiers declared in 1925 that the feebleminded "are controlled entirely by the lower passions causing them to be more prolific than the normal person" and that "80 percent of the feeble-minded are born of feeble-minded parents." His solution:

> There will be a bill introduced in the present Legislature which in our opinion will greatly lessen this burden, the bill permitting sterilization under proper restrictions.
>
> The operation is very slight, produces no harmful results, the patient suffers no pain or discomforts.

Asserting that "we do not know enough about heredity to take the step of sterilizing inmates of institutions" and that "the principle is all wrong," Dr. Forrest C. Tyson, superintendent of the Augusta State Hospital, appeared alone before the Judiciary committee in opposition to a measure which would regulate sterilization of inmates in State institutions.

—Lewiston Daily Sun, *March 12, 1931*

> It is better for all the world, if, instead of waiting to execute degenerate offspring for crime, society can prevent those who are manifestly unfit from continuing their kind.
>
> —*Associate Justice Oliver Wendell Holmes in a U.S. Supreme Court decision upholding a Virginia sterilization law*

These, in brief, are a few reasons why I am in favor of sterilization for both male and female in certain cases of feeble mindedness.

It is a means to prevent reproduction of all moral imbeciles; to permanently improve the human race, to enforce in a simple way, sound, decent and efficient human beings . . . and it is the most humane way.

Later that year, the legislature approved such a bill. It was not enough for everybody, said a worried writer in an October 1925 edition of the *Lewiston Journal*:

There are many men, of conscience and of courage; Christian and Gentle; who look on the idiots at Pownal, far worse than animals, for animals have their own powers intact, and wonder if a certain form of peaceful extermination were not better. You may shudder at this expression and no one makes it—certainly not we—as an advocate of the policy. We merely state what has been pondered over by others. The Swine which were possessed of demons as related in the Scriptures were more respectably off in this scheme of a world, than these poor travesties of human-beings.

We have a law that permits the State to sterilize these people. But it is so hedged about, that it is little used. There are so many permissions and writings and attestations to be made that it is too roundabout to do much good.

In 1932, Vosburgh summarized the effects of the law at the school:

The policy of this school in following out the intent of the law has been one of selective sterilization, using conservative judgment in recommending the operative procedure, and has been quite satisfactory. The Pownal State School is custodian of all papers and records of eugenic sterilization performed under these acts, and up to the present time there have been thirty-four operations. Of these, twenty-one have been performed upon those committed to the School for care. Consideration for sterilization is

On Dec. 3, in the evening, at the end of the moving picture entertainment, one of the films broke, and took fire, but it was extinguished promptly, causing only some discomfort to the men by reason of gas formed by the extinguishing fluid, but no damage was done excepting for a short length of film.

—*Dr. Stephen E. Vosburgh, monthly report to the commissioner of Health and Welfare, 1932*

given at the time of discharge of every case, and in general those who are fitted by training to be at least partly self-supporting are recommended for the operative procedure. This policy has been well accepted by those interested in taking their relatives home, as they have realized the situation and have in many instances taken the initiative in making the request.

Much writing of the time stressed the sensational and called for strong and repressive measures such as sterilization. But much energy at the campus was going to more positive purpose—expanding the plant and improving the programs within it.

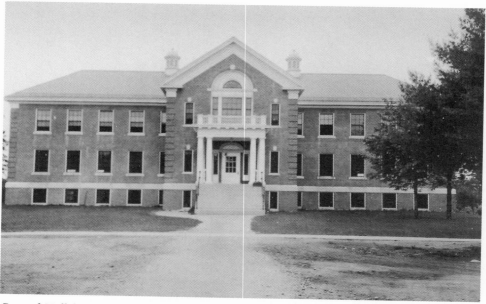

Pownal Hall (courtesy of the New Gloucester Historical Society)

One of the assistants in the engineer's department will be assigned the duty each Sunday morning of winding, setting, and regulating the clocks in the Central Group, to correspond with the office and engine room clocks. The matrons and those in charge of the various buildings where clocks are in operation shall check the time of their clock daily with the whistle signals. If there is any great variance the engineer should be notified, so that corrections can be made.

—*Dr. Stephen E. Vosburgh, general bulletin, April 24, 1930*

A New Name and New Buildings

Some supporters of the school objected that its name was too negative. Vosburgh acted on the complaint in 1925, saying, "In consequence of the almost universal objection of friends and relatives of those sent here, and also because of the modern tendency to eliminate distressing terms, I recommend that the Legislature be requested to change the name of the Maine School for Feeble-Minded to Pownal State School." Maine's legislators agreed, and the change became official before the year was out. Nobody seemed concerned that most of the school was in New Gloucester, not Pownal. The name worked well because the West Pownal post office was nearby.

Signs declaring the new name welcomed visitors to a place already changed from the way Vosburgh had first found it. Yarmouth Hall, a dormitory for girls, had opened in 1921 as Dirigo House (a name that would go to a new superintendent's house in 1929). The electrification of campus and farm buildings was continuing. A new powerhouse and laundry had been erected. And Pownal Hall, a building for boys, was close to completion.

The school at this point was devising its physical plant as it went, working loosely on an early plan created by its first chief engineer. In 1921, Vosburgh asked for ideas from the Olmsted Brothers of Brookline, Massachusetts, the firm founded by Frederick Law Olmsted, who had won great fame for New York's Central Park and other creations before his death in 1903. Carl Rust Parker, a member of the firm, visited the school in 1921 and reported disdainfully in his personal notes that

> *. . . because of the fact that the original plan was very badly conceived and because of the fact that there has been more or less of a hit or miss arrangement in locating new buildings since the school started, the whole*

> If in the [hospital elevator car] when it stops, if opposite a landing, open the door; or, if midway, press the emergency button, wait a few minutes, then try to start it again.
> —*Dr. Stephen E. Vosburgh, notice to staff, November 21, 1931*

proposition is somewhat of a mess and it will never be possible to make it a particularly attractive institution. . . .

Parker would eventually submit his own proposals, but they would not control the school's development. Vosburgh later reported that they had been merged with earlier strategies and some additional later ideas to form a new working concept.

Not everybody felt as Parker did about the plant. The new brick buildings reminded some visitors of a small country college, and the *Portland Sunday Telegram* proudly presented photographs of them in an impressive layout appearing in July 1927.

But for those on the campus, there was little time to sit around and stare at the new structures. For one thing, other buildings needed repair, such as the central kitchen, where half the ceiling fell, wounding two employees, in 1924. And growth demanded more growth. There was much to be done, and the legislature was not always generous with funds.

In 1925, as Pownal Hall was about to provide 150 new beds for males, Vosburgh asked for a staff increase of a physician, a music teacher, a first-grade teacher, a stenographer, a plumber, a chef, a serving-room attendant, a night watchman, a night telephone operator, a laundress, two nurses, seven day attendants, and two night attendants. The governor and council approved these increases, even though the legislature had been going through a frugal period for a couple of sessions. A few years later, in 1931, the new Hedin Hospital opened to serve the residents of the Pownal school and some other state institutions as well. Hedin gave the school such long-awaited facilities as an emergency operating room; a dentist's space; an eye, ear, nose, and throat room; a pharmacy; and a four-section mortuary "equipped with Frigidaire cooling, with autopsy table and equipment." But now Vosburgh had new cause to worry, and he did:

The rooming quarters of employees present a serious problem. We have taken all available rooms for use, including rooms assigned to inmates, reception rooms, rooms in basement previously used for [a] dentist. This was necessary because of the increased number of employees due to the opening of the hospital building and the Legislature not passing the request for three officers' cottages, which would have relieved another building and permitted a readjustment. It is absolutely necessary that something be done, and the only alternative is the temporary use of a basement room in the hospital building for an isolation ward, this room having been built for lavatory purposes, and using the two small rooms vacated by this arrangement for employees. This is undesirable because they are located in the basement, but we have no alternative.

Programs

The institution also needed new school buildings, the superintendent said in 1932. "The academic, physical and manual training are now carried on in basement rooms or attics which are unfitted for such use." But despite the limited space, training efforts were intense.

Special effort is made to assign each individual to the particular school or training group to which he is fitted and from which he would receive the most benefit. The training is carried to the limit of the capacity of each individual, to make him or her as nearly self-supporting as possible, therefore making discharge of selected cases possible.

The programs were productive, too. In fact, the school's inmates repaired and produced much of the equipment and clothing used at the school. In one year the boys in the industrial arts school made 80 articles, valued at $89.02, and the girls made 193 articles, valued at $177.54. Inmates in the manual training department produced 1,538 articles, with a value of $3,792.11. During the same year, food produced by the school's farms had more than half the value of the food used by the

I really in a way made it so I could enjoy myself here, because I felt that was the necessary thing, to make the best of it, and I did. I got the best out of it. I had a good education. The teachers taught us well, taught us how to live with people, and how to get along, and how to be honest. They read the Bible story to us every morning. I attribute my love to those teachers. They're gone now, and I'll never forget them.

—*Charles O. Wyman, recalling his days at the Pownal State School, in* Making the Best of It, *a film created by Bates College students to tell his story after his return in 1989*

Through the years Pownal has been the meeting place of several couples who later married. The newspapers of 1930, for example, carried the account of the marriage of Dr. Harris M. Carey, physician at the School, and Miss Anna B. Marriner, superintendent of nurses at the School. This was not the first couple to meet and marry while working here, and it certainly wasn't the last.
—Pineland Observer, *March and April 1968*

dietary department. "All milk, cream, one-half of butter, veal, pork, one-third of the beef, fowl, chicken and broilers, eggs, and vegetables and garden truck are produced by this department," said the annual report for the period.

The school often displayed its products in local fairs and exhibits, and a news report after the 1936 Spring Hobby and Handicraft Exposition in Lewiston said that "the State School at Pownal had an outstanding exhibit of work of the patients there, unique in many ways. Furniture, rope rugs, hooked and braided rugs, embroidery and other articles were original in design and craftsmanship."

The director of education at the time supervised academic, industrial, musical, physical training, special schools, and monthly dances for employees. The faculty included academic, industrial arts, and physical education teachers. Outside

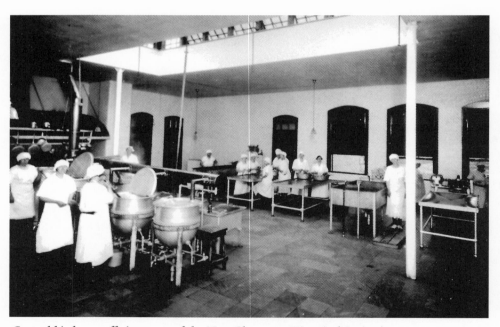

Central kitchen staff (courtesy of the New Gloucester Historical Society)

class, inmates could participate in Campfire Girls and Boy Scout activities, and the Boy Scout troop drew much attention for presentations it gave off campus. At a jamboree at Portland's City Hall, the boys performed before 3,000 spectators and a news account approved: "One of the most interesting features was the Indian ceremonial as enacted by carefully drilled scouts from the Pownal State School. These boys, garbed in the savage costumes, reproduced the Indian songs and dances and 'brought down the house' with their performance."

Formal photographs of the Boy Scout and Campfire Girls groups stand in sharp contrast to press reports of the feebleminded as immoral degenerates. So do reports of social and recreational activities at the school. One was "Deacon Dubbs," a drama coached by Mrs. Vosburgh and presented for the amusement of the children. "There was a splendid ukulele chorus that sang old time songs," said the *Lewiston Evening Journal*, as well as a "hick orchestra," dances, and vocal duets. "The program was enjoyed immensely by the children and well might it have been enjoyed by anyone."

The drama's participants included Louisa Lowe, the teenage daughter of the school's chief farmer, Christopher Lowe. Louisa often played piano to accompany the silent movies shown to staff and inmates on a regular basis, and she played with the school choir. "The kids loved to sing," she would remember many years later as she approached the age of ninety. "They had a very patient director who taught them the music and they were really very good." Now Louisa Lowe Bishop, the former accompanist also recalled with pleasure the school's many celebrations, on the Fourth of July, for example, and at Christmas, when her father would appear from a fireplace dressed as Santa Claus.

Louisa Lowe encountered the larger world's fear of the feebleminded on at least one occasion. When her own high school was closed for a day, she went to visit a friend's school. The girl told her classmates that Louisa came from the School for Feeble-Minded, and that was the end of Louisa's chance to make new friends.

Dr. and Mrs. Stephen E. Vosburgh of the Pownal State School were at home informally to the school family on Sunday afternoon from 3 to 6 o'clock when a large number availed themselves of this opportunity to greet the host and hostess, and to view the superintendent's new house, which has been completed recently.

Modern in every detail, this new house of Colonial type with its spacious rooms and sun parlor, all closely carried out in attractive color scheme, is a valuable addition to the State School.

—Kennebec Journal, *February 28, 1929*

"They wouldn't have a thing to do with me," she said, the memory still smarting. "They were too scared of me."

Louisa and other staff family members did not intermingle frequently with inmates, but still she saw a different side of life. There was Johnny, for example, the "huge man who was assigned to do chores for our family. He was so big that the side he was on in the Fourth of July rope pull always won. I remember that every Sunday he made ice cream in a hand-cranked mixer, and he always got the first bowl. And it was a big bowl." Johnny "adored our family," Bishop remembered. He was "broken hearted when my father and mother retired," but he was able to visit the Lowes occasionally on their nearby farm.

Johnny was not the only inmate to spend time in local homes. Many were hired for two dollars a day plus a huge midday meal, the boys to do farmwork and the girls to do housekeeping. "The kids just loved the weeding and other farmwork," both at the school and outside it, Bishop remembered. "They thought it was great fun."

Superintendent Vosburgh had a boy named Charlie assigned to his own family, according to Bishop. Charlie was once mistaken for the doctor as he left the doctor's car, and he played the role happily, creating a story that swept through the campus and amused the staff greatly.

Placing the mothers of Maine in the same department and under the same control as murderers is a proposal that may well give Maine citizens pause. Yet this is the proposal of the administrative code.

For good measure there are thrown in the tubercular and the insane, the delinquent and the feeble-minded, the Indians and the orphans, the veterans and their dependents. One department that embraces all the criminals and widowed mothers of Maine and their dependent children and all the health work of sundry kinds in which the state or any town is engaged seems both unprecedented and unwise.

—*Former governor Ralph O. Brewster, speaking against Governor Gardiner's proposed reorganization of 1931*

We have a notion that if a general oversight of all beneficent institutions were to be placed under the direction of such a man as Dr. Vosburgh, no mother would be confused with a murderer; and no murderer would be mistaken for a mother.

—Lewiston Evening Journal *responding to Governor Brewster, May 15, 1931*

Modernization

The school changed frequently with the times, and in 1931 the showing of silent films came to an end. Nobody was making them anymore, and Vosburgh had to seek funds for a new sound projector.

That was only one of many signs of change. The previous year, the doctor had issued a memo saying that the "large number of privately owned automobiles now housed on the State grounds necessitate issuing rules and regulations." Garage space would be provided only at the discretion of the superintendent, he declared. No supplies for washing private vehicles would be issued by the school, and "it is forbidden that inmates be recruited for work on privately owned cars."

Another memo came from Vosburgh in 1931:

> Those enjoying radio receptions sometimes forget that others living in the same building are annoyed by having the reception extremely loud. Likewise, it is expected that employees who are on duty (even though living in quarters where, perhaps, some of their work is detailed) will not use the machines during their working hours. It seems necessary to ask that when the radio is used at proper times, it is to be modulated so that it will not annoy others.

State government was changing, too. On January 1, 1932, a major restructuring occurred, effected through a fresh administrative code proposed and championed by Governor William Tudor Gardiner. The board of trustees that had run the school since its founding was out, with a new state commissioner of Health and Welfare taking many of its powers—despite loud protests about the idea of giving a single individual control over both health programs and criminal institutions. Superintendent Vosburgh was mentioned in the press as a likely candidate for the position, but when he said he was not interested, Gardiner gave it to George W. Leadbetter on a temporary basis.

Even the language of institutions such as Pownal was changing. A *Kennebec Journal* reporter heard Vosburgh address some Kiwanians in March 1931 and duly gave this report:

> The term "feeble-minded" has been abandoned for the broader term of "sub-normal," said the doctor. Many of those cared for in institutions actually have superior intelligences, but are so lacking in other qualities as to be unable to live normally. The Pownal institution, commonly termed a school for feeble-minded, is in reality a school for feeble personalities, it was explained.

> In January of 1927 the school employees staged a mock trial for the patients in which a young lady obtained a breach of promise settlement for a broken engagement. Other entertainment was provided by two members of the staff, Curtis Hughes and Dr. Nessib S. Kupelian. . . . Dr. Vosburgh played foreman of the jury.
>
> —Pineland Observer, *special edition, 1968*

The reporter did not say why the article itself continued to use the term "feeble-minded" in the wrong name it gave to Vosburgh's place of work, the "State School for Feeble Minded at Pownal" (or why it spelled the doctor's name without the "h"). But the paper's failure to abandon "feeble-minded" was not uncommon. That term would appear in occasional news reports and various school documents for years.

Another word falling into disuse was "inmates." Although it too would continue cropping up from time to time, "patients" would increasingly replace it.

Getting Out

School programs, Christmas parties, and movie nights probably sounded good to many Maine citizens who read reports about the school in the 1920s and 1930s. Some of them responded with contributions intended to improve life at the school even more, and the superintendent's annual reports regularly listed gifts such as clothing, postcards, and candy that had arrived during the year.

But neither programs nor gifts were enough to make all the patients happy with their fate. Those behind the school's locked doors knew that they might well stay for life. Some had been sent primarily because of behavioral problems or family poverty, but they were soon tested, classified as feebleminded, and made to remain. True, a few were judged to be improved and were released each year, but they were a small minority. In the year ending June 30, 1933, twenty-eight patients left; that was only 3 percent of the population, which was 809 at year's close. Most residents could imagine nothing brighter than lifelong confinement at the school, and more than a few who hated that vision did their best to get out. Somehow they disagreed with the assessment of a man who visited the school in 1927 and reported that everyone there "was better off than ever before in his or her life, there could be no doubt about that."

The newspapers told frequent stories of escape and recapture, arrest and return to Pownal The problem troubled Vosburgh, who suggested to his board in 1925 that one reason was the presence of delinquents in the school population:

Brunswick, Dec. 9—Walter Haney, 21, walked into the Brunswick police station today, told Chief William B. Edwards that he escaped from the State School at Pownal three years ago and that after traveling about the country, he preferred to spend a prospective tough winter back at the school. The Pownal authorities were notified and will come here for Haney Thursday.

—Portland Press Herald, *December 10, 1931*

I wish to report the unusual number of escapes which we are having, from the newly admitted cases. It has been our experience that whenever a large group of new boys are received, escapes increase until they have become adjusted. In no instance have these escapees been out over a few hours. During the past month we have had eight such escapes. . . . Eventually, it is my opinion, as expressed in several annual reports, that if this institution is to care for defective delinquents, a separate building will be necessary which will be under more strict oversight. Most other states have separate institutions for such cases.

The superintendent remarked on the problem again in 1931:

We had two group escapes of boys, in one instance six, but all have been returned and were out only a short time without any harmful effects. The unrest, which is particularly prevalent among the boys, requires very careful supervision, and it is almost impossible to prevent an occasional escape. This unrest seems to be prevalent in all institutions and is evidently the reaction against control and supervision.

It was during Vosburgh's tenure that the most famous of the school's escapees left the grounds. He was Charles O. Wyman, who had arrived at the school on June

I looked up at those big buildings and I thought it was a prison or something and it scared me. . . . The matron came out and she grabbed me and started screeching and hollering and I thought there was something the matter with her mind.

—*Charles O. Wyman, recalling his arrival at the Pownal State School, in* Making the Best of It, *a film created by Bates College students to tell his story after his return in 1989*

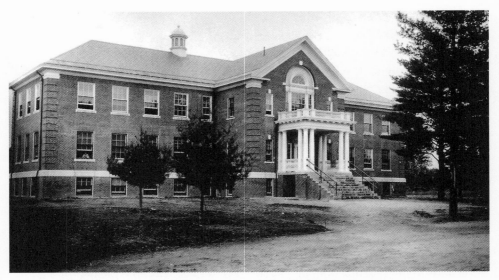

Yarmouth Hall (courtesy of the New Gloucester Historical Society)

22, 1920, at the age of nine. Charlie was far from feebleminded and far from pleased with the Pownal institution, where he was soon locked alone in a room for several months while recovering from tuberculosis. In 1929, after two failed attempts, he ran off to hide in a nearby barn, then made his way home to his family in the Bangor area. The next decades would be good to him. He found work even during the Depression, married, served in the army during the Second World War, had children, gave his name to a trout fly he created, and then surprised the world by returning to the school as an old man and telling his story again and again to a delighted press.

He explained that he had been sent to the school by the town of Troy after fire burned the family home and his parents were arrested for failure to nurture their children. How was life at the school? a reporter asked. "Did anybody tuck you in at night?"

"They tucked you in with a strap," Wyman said. And they used the strap on inmates, he reported, after first making them lie in a bathtub with ice packs to chill the skin so the strap marks wouldn't show.

Another inmate of that period would report in the 1990s that scalding had sometimes been used as a punishment. Another would remember an attendant who struck with a rubber hose, and a second who carried brass knuckles. There was talk about shaving heads of inmates who attempted escape or showed too much interest in patients of the opposite gender. Such punishments were outside the stated policy of Pownal, and some contemporaries, such as Louisa Bishop,

The forms of discipline in use in this institution are as follows:
1. Standing during a meal.
2. Loss of dessert.
3. Bread and water for a meal.
4. Standing during a meal with bread and milk.
5. Sitting at matron's doors or in corner.
6. Sending to bed.
7. Sending to bed with bread and milk.
8. Attending chapel or entertainment in work clothes.
9. Non-attendance at one or more entertainments.
10. Wearing of a camisole [straitjacket].

All correction must be administered by the matrons with the approval of the physician and a full report shall be made on the Matron's Daily Report sheet in that section designated.

No correction of any kind should be administered but for the child's good. We are so largely creatures of impulse that vindictiveness is likely to add force, if not injustice, to the discipline administered on the spur of the moment.

A distinction should be made between correction and medical treatment. . . .

Institutions are occasionally subjected to scrutiny because of some indiscretion of an employee. We have been particularly free from such complaints, and let us continue by example and instruction of the less experienced employees to play fair with the children.

—Dr. Stephen E. Vosburgh, bulletin, April 28, 1930

doubted the stories about them. "I have heard them," she said, "but I don't think they are right."

Whatever the punishments used at Pownal, they wouldn't keep everybody there. Another escapee who made the news was Mrs. Eleanor M. Chase Libby. Her attorney later claimed that Eleanor Chase had been sentenced as a minor to the state school for girls in Hallowell, then illegally transferred to Pownal without a hearing. She and a companion escaped in December 1936 and were taken in by Archie Cushman, a male school employee who lived in Yarmouth. By the time the police caught up with them, Eleanor Chase had married another man, Harry E. Libby. The authorities declared that the marriage was illegal and did not count because the woman was feebleminded. They leveled charges against Cushman and

Libby, and returned the women to Pownal. Mrs. Libby then petitioned for her free-dom, and at a court hearing complained that she had been disciplined by being placed in a straitjacket a short time before the hearing. "If she is feeble-minded, so am I," her attorney told the court. The hearing before a Supreme Court justice ended with a compromise in which Mrs. Libby dropped her complaint and the school released her.

Some of those who left the school by more legitimate means than escape had to pay a higher, more dangerous price than shaved heads: surgical sterilization. "You may leave," the school told them in effect, "but only if you first agree to the operation." Two young women who accepted the bargain in order to rejoin their family in 1932 were twins, Mabel and Mildred Wahl. The operation went poorly for Mildred, who died the next day of a blood clot in her lung. Mabel's surgery was also difficult, but she survived and left the school for a long life outside it.

Staying on Board

Superintendent Vosburgh gave great energy to keeping not just inmates but also staff members at the school. Some individuals and even families gave faithful serv-ice for decades. Louisa Lowe Bishop would follow her parents into employment there, for instance. And her daughter would come after her, then three of her daughter's four children. But for others the stay was short.

State pay was not generous, and the work could be difficult. Staff members lived at the school, far from urban pleasures. From the beginning, turnover was high. The number of employees at the school averaged 53 in 1919, when Vosburgh arrived; the number who left that year was 94. The superintendent took a system-atic approach to improving conditions and satisfying his workers. In 1927, the average number of employees, 114, was larger than the number who left, 87. By 1933, the *Lewiston Journal* could offer this description of the changes:

> . . . As Dr. Vosburgh said, "Unless there is an acceptable administra-tion policy with fixed rules, a definite delegation of authority, considera-tion in sickness, a reasonably appetizing diet, clean living quarters and reasonable hours of work and off duty, the salary is of little interest."

It is requested and directed that the wearing of abbreviated costumes such as "shorts" on these grounds be prohibited. Exception to this rule is made for those who direct or take part in class work during such class hours as approved.

—*Dr. Stephen E. Vosburgh, notice to staff, July 12, 1934*

With this data, Dr. Vosburgh set about to change conditions. . . .
Thirteen departments were organized, with designations of the responsi-
bility of each head and of employee associates. Then came recognized hol-
idays, a sickness policy, food menu planning and table service under care
of a dietician, livable dining-rooms with small tables, a system of service,
a six-day week, with daily hours off to even work to 8 or 8¹/₂ hours, and
an average salary increase from $7.53 a week in 1914 to $13.66 in 1925.
Present employees number 157, and they are well trained and efficient and
comfortably situated.

In the 1930s, of course, the Depression might have helped keep staff members
in their jobs. There was little work available elsewhere, and turnover continued to
decrease even after the state cut salaries and forced employees to take two-week
vacations without pay.

Troubling Times

Staff retention was not the only way the Depression affected the Pownal State
School. The legislature was trying to trim budgets everywhere. Per capita weekly
expenses had reached $6.92 in 1931. They decreased to $6.75 in 1932. Individual
families also suffered. Some could not afford to bring their children home even
when the school would release them, and requests to do so ended for a time.
Vosburgh spoke about this in a 1932 report:

A remarkable situation regarding requests for discharge is at present
evident. Whereas it has been usual to receive requests for the dismissal of
five to twelve cases, it is probable that the general conditions are such that
relatives are not seeking to assume responsibility.

The school continued to grow just the same. After all, the waiting lists were
still there, fed by other institutions with inmates they deemed subnormal, by
families and town officials seeking to place the impoverished, and by courts dealing with young offenders. In 1937, the school opened two new dormitories plus
additions to the laundry and nurses' home. The school could accommodate 1,120
patients. But this was still not enough. "It is obvious that overcrowding must again
begin almost immediately," said a January edition of the *Lewiston Sun Journal* in
a report on $2 million worth of construction at various Maine institutions:

Altho the greatest increase in capacity is at the Pownal State School—
home for feeble minded—where 320 additional beds have been provided,
it will not do away with the waiting list for, at this time, there are more
than 400 in the State who should be sent there.

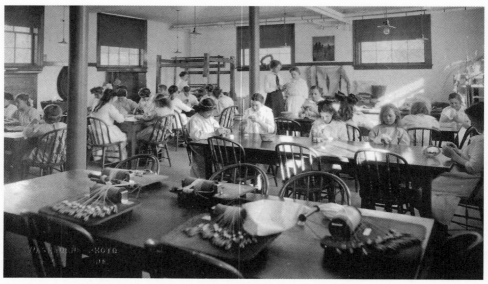

Manual training class (courtesy of the New Gloucester Historical Society)

World war was fast approaching. Human, state, and national resources would soon be diverted again from institutions such as the Pownal State School, creating critical problems.

But Vosburgh would not live to see or solve them. He was stricken in August 1937 by heart problems and died on December 24. Said the *Portland Press Herald* the following day:

> *The untimely death of Dr. Stephen E. Vosburgh clouds Christmas Day for his wide circle of friends and is a serious blow to the State of Maine which he had served for a quarter of a century. In all the institutions of which he had been a part he had made an admirable record. The condition and operation of the Pownal State School, with which he had most recently been associated as head, have long been acclaimed a triumph for skillfully wise management.*

> December 24, Dr. Vosburgh passed away very suddenly this morning at Dirigo House at about 2:45 o'clock, of a coronary occlusion. Flags were hung at half mast, at the order of Dr. Kupelian, with the approval of Dr. Hanscom. The children had their Christmas trees in the afternoon and received their presents, but all entertainments were cancelled.
>
> —*Superintendent's monthly report, December 1937*

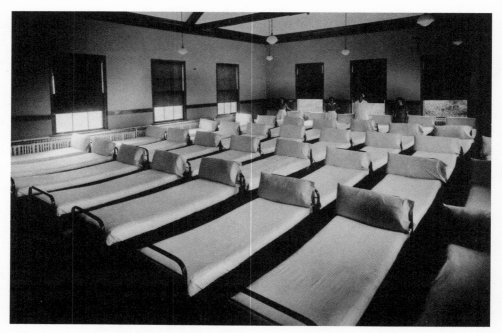

Beds in New Gloucester Hall (courtesy of the New Gloucester Historical Society)

The Kupelian Years: 1938–1953 | 3

You can no more win a war than you can win an earthquake.

—Jeannette Rankin

Aquick glance shows the Kupelian era at Pownal State School as a series of sporadic and scorching flare-ups, both figurative and literal. A deeper look reveals it as a period of painful crunch, a time when the demand for services increased dramatically while the means to provide them decreased dangerously.

Americans might have fought the Second World War for the most part on foreign soil, but its victims were everywhere, including the Pownal State School in Maine. The problem was not that people didn't care, but that their care was stretched thin to the point of near rupture. The Second World War was a mad international crisis diverting from Pownal not just the state's attention but its human, fiscal, and material resources as well. And that war was not the only challenge of the era; the Great Depression that preceded it plus the inflation and the Korean War that followed it all took their toll.

> Harry S. Coombs, Architect, Lewiston, passed away this morning at 3 A.M., after an illness of some months. . . . Mr. Coombs had been connected with the School as Architect since the very early days of the Institution and had helped design nearly all of the brick buildings at this school, the firm name being Coombs & Gibbs and later Coombs & Harriman.
>
> —*Dr. N. S. Kupelian, monthly report, May 31, 1939*

> The children have shown great appreciation of the six new radios which have been purchased and installed in accordance with former arrangements. Even some of the lower grade children can enjoy the music and other programs. The outcome has been remarkable for two reasons: one is that the children are having great enjoyment, as before stated, listening to the programs; and the second is that it has eliminated the noise and confusion so that many of the children sit by the hour and listen to the music and entertainment, and afterwards some of the low grade children are heard humming the tunes.
>
> *—Dr. N. S. Kupelian, monthly report, May 31, 1938*

The New Superintendent

Many readers of Maine newspapers already knew something of the new superintendent. Dr. Nessib S. Kupelian had been at the school for sixteen years and was both assistant superintendent and director of Hedin Hospital at the time of his predecessor's death. The *Lewiston Evening Journal* considered Kupelian a good man and said so in a description of the hospital's first fourteen months, published in November 1932:

> *Seeing Dr. Kupelian, one finds a kindly type of physician, gentle of soul and well-trained for his work, with only words of praise for all his assistants. . . .*
>
> *"We have had in this period," he explained, in answer to questions, "some 789 patients, so that the beds have been full all the time. In other words, the hospital is used to capacity. Some are coming in and others going out, and the cases range, as in any hospital, from slight troubles like cuts and bruises to surgical work of minor and major character. . . ."*
>
> *New is the work for crippled children, 12 of them having been operated on to relieve their condition. . . .*
>
> *Another new development is trepanning the skull, to relieve pressure on the brain, and thereby restore the individual's faculties, which have been affected by artificial pressure, as from some accident. . . .*

Kupelian shared much with his predecessors. He was a medical doctor, and would continue performing medical duties, including surgery, throughout his superintendency. Very much at the center of the school's operation, he was viewed by both the public and his staff as the school's voice as well as its leader in matters

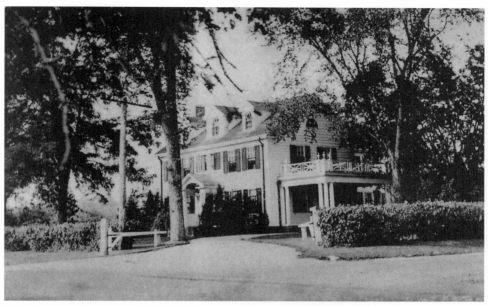

Superintendent's house (courtesy of the New Gloucester Historical Society)

large and small. So many people relied on his office for direction that he felt the need to issue this written notice in 1947:

> *It is becoming so that employees are calling the Superintendent's Secretary for everything, to make inquiries or to ask questions of the Superintendent. These calls have increased so that it practically takes most of the time of the Secretary. Many of these questions should be taken up directly with the Departmental Head or with the Financial Office. Matters which are very important can be brought to the Superintendent through*

It has come to my attention that gambling is going on among the male employees and the boys are participating in the games. It is quite evident the boys are given money by the employees and sometimes articles owned by the State are purchased from the boys. Gambling is not only against the laws of Maine but against the rules of the Institution. Any further evidence of this practice or any employee purchasing State property from a patient or giving them money without going through the regular channels will be subject for immediate dismissal.

—*Dr. N. S. Kupelian, notice, November 24, 1947*

[Mrs. K. C.], relative of [M. N.], has signed a paper, giving consent to [M.'s] eugenic sterilization, and [M]. herself desires it. Her father has been sent a paper to sign, in case he consents to the voluntary operation. If the necessary consent is given, it is recommended that this operation be performed, with a view to [M's] discharge following convalescence, into the custody of [Mrs. C]. [M.] is now 21 years old and her last test classified her as a moron . . . It is believed that with supervision [M.] may be able to get along in the community, as she seems to have a sense of right and wrong, and is sociable and kind-hearted. Although handicapped physically, she is able to do some domestic work. The State would have to bear the expense of the operation.
—*Dr. N. S. Kupelian, monthly report, March 31, 1939*

the regular channels or by making an appointment with the Superintendent for a personal interview. I would therefore ask that the employees do not make unnecessary calls to the Superintendent or the Superintendent's Office.

Like Vosburgh before him, Kupelian was a forceful advocate of sterilization. In 1941 he supported a bill introduced to the legislature by Senator Neil S. Bishop of Bowdoinham, a measure that would establish a State Board of Eugenics empowered to order sterilization of Maine "defectives" outside of institutions. Bishop was a strong friend of the school, and his opinions were often strong, too. "In work with animals and plants," he said in explanation of his bill, "we have spent millions to improve the breed, the strain and the families. Virtually nothing has been done to improve the human race." But Bishop's bill was heartily condemned by others, including the Roman Catholic bishop of Portland, who called it "vicious and un-Christian." The Senate rejected it by a vote of 28 to 4. Sterilization could and would continue at the school for some years to come, but demands to expand it began to fade from the press, at least in part, no doubt, because of increasing reaction to grotesque Nazi attempts at improving the Aryan race and eliminating others.

Kupelian also continued his predecessors' call for continuing institutional growth, telling the Auburn and Lewiston Kiwanis Club in 1940 that the school's accommodations for 1,100 defective persons should be expanded to care for 7,900 more, the *Lewiston Evening Journal* reported.

The Yellow Soap Flare-up

The job came with rewards. Community respect was one, and the superintendent's house was another. Kupelian's son Phillip had been born in the Morse House, another staff residence on the campus. He was thirteen when the family moved into Dirigo House, the superintendent's home, and he remembered it well more than sixty years later. "Of all the times I ever moved I think I liked that one best," he said. "They really built that house well. It was a wonderful home."

But there were challenges, too, major challenges, and one of the first to engage the new superintendent hit the news in March 1938. The headlines from the *Maine Sunday Telegram* were large, in 72-point type: "Charges of Neglect At Pownal State School To Be Filed, Connolly Says." Connolly was a local attorney and former Superior Court judge. He promised further investigation, but his opening salvo offered plenty for the paper to report:

> *Specific allegations upon which he has already heard enough to give strong reason for bringing charges, Mr. Connolly said, include lack of adequate winter clothing, scarcity of disinfectants needed in such an institution, improper ventilation through efforts to conserve on heat, and lack of bath soap, resulting in an epidemic of severe skin rash.*
>
> *Many of the inmates are still wearing summer underwear, he declared he had been informed by employees in a position to know of such conditions. Outer clothing is dilapidated and ragged, having been repaired as much as possible, and one boy, a few days ago, was found without any underwear. The result has been, he said, that the hospital has been filled to capacity much of the time with inmates suffering from severe colds and bronchial troubles.*

It has become necessary again to call the attention of employees to children's personal correspondence. Each child is permitted to write only one letter each week and it must be to a relative, if not, an approved person. Matrons should instruct children not to write unreasonably long and begging letters. An increasing number of children are asking relatives to write to the Superintendent for them to go on vacation. This practice must be discouraged. The granting of vacations or visits depends upon mental progress, behavior and home surroundings of each case. It is only when these requirements are satisfactory that a visit will be considered.

—*Dr. N. S. Kupelian, notice, April 8, 1940*

> When the doctor came into the room we had to stand up. Isn't that crazy?
>
> When we ate we stood up and said grace. Then we had to eat in fifteen minutes. If we didn't finish they took the food away. Isn't that crazy?
>
> If we talked too loud they made us walk around the room. Isn't that crazy?
>
> If you walked outdoors, you couldn't go alone. Isn't that crazy?
>
> If you spoke to a girl they put you in a room. Isn't that crazy? That's foolish business. That's crazy, that is.
>
> *—Edward B., who was placed at the Pownal State School in 1937 after being falsely accused of theft. He stayed for twenty-six years and shared his memory of them in November 2000*

Within the last few days, according to the information collected by Mr. Connolly, the supply of bath soap has been exhausted. Inmates have been obliged to use ordinary "yellow" scrubbing soap, which has caused many cases of severe skin rash. Saturday night was "bath night" and it was declared there was no soap of any kind left for use in the Saturday night ablutions.

Supported by Dr. George W. Leadbetter, who headed the supervising Department of Health and Welfare in Augusta, Kupelian responded on Sunday, March 6, calling the charges "an attack," describing them as "absolutely false," and saying he "would welcome an investigation of the school by anyone at any time." On Monday, Governor Lewis O. Barrows ordered a probe by Leadbetter and other state officials, who would travel to the school and check conditions on Wednesday. By the end of the week, the *Portland Press Herald* announced in 24-point type that "No Grounds Exist for Complaints At Pownal, Committee Tells Governor." Connolly, according to the committee, "stated that he did not make the charges and was not sponsoring the same, that he was not interested beyond the point of bringing the matter to the attention of the Governor." The information actually came from Dr. J. R. Andrews, who had recently been dismissed by Kupelian on charges of "continued intoxication, insubordination and neglect of duty." The headlines remained small as successive stories reported Andrews's demand for an impartial hearing, the scheduling of such a hearing, and Andrews's failure to attend it. At the end of the month the state personnel board declared Andrews's dismissal to be justified. Any damage inflicted on the school appeared temporary.

A Year Later

Throughout his superintendency, Kupelian would worry about how few people visited and understood Pownal State School. Augusta's *Kennebec Journal* for February 8, 1939, carried his remarks on that matter at the beginning of a newspaper article he wrote each year describing Pownal to readers:

> *It is surprising to know that very few of the citizens of Maine have any conception of the work accomplished in this school, which is one of the three largest institutions in the State of Maine. The purpose behind its establishment and development is to provide custodial care, education and training for mentally subnormal human beings of the State. The institution is a small village with several departments through which the various activities are carried on. Since its inception in 1908, the school has grown so that it has at present a population of 1073 patients with 200 employees. There are 51 buildings, some small but others are beautiful permanent constructions. The buildings are located in three groups: a central one where the administrative activities and the academic and industrial training are concentrated; and two farm colonies for 60 boys each, located about one-half mile from the central group. A complete water system consists of three pumps of 400 and 250 gallons a minute. A central heating and power plant furnishes steam and generates electricity, supplying with power the central kitchen, laundry, carpenter shop, and the pumping station; and lighting to all groups.*

Complete with an aerial photograph of the campus, the long article included a history of the school, a lengthy account of its social and training activities, and notes about the employment of patients:

> *Planning, preparing and serving a well balanced diet with proper caloric values for nearly 1300 people is a big task. There are in the institution a good many crippled and paralytic children with very feeble digestion, who require special diets. Also, there is a large number of patients with epileptic convulsions whose dietary regimen needs close supervision. There*

Found guilty of delinquency, a 13-year-old Augusta youth was sentenced Friday to the Pownal School by Judge Arthur A. Hebert.

Police asserted the charge arose out of the theft of a car belonging to Commissioner Harry O. Page of the Health and Welfare Department.

—Kennebec Journal, *February 2, 1945*

Hitler, described as "the arch dictator," was defined as a neurotic by Dr. N. S. Kupelian, superintendent of the State School at Pownal, at the luncheon meeting today of the Portland Kiwanis Club at the Lafayette Hotel.

Dr. Kupelian pointed out that the German Fuehrer as a neurotic is headed for the hospital for the insane, if he is not already there, "and the sooner the better," the speaker added.

—Portland Evening Express, *May 25, 1943*

are about 70 inmate girls employed in the central kitchen, where they receive instructions about cooking, serving meals and waiting at tables, etc. . . .

There are about 60 of the male patients receiving very helpful instructions on the farm. It is expected that some of these boys can be gainfully employed on a farm when the opportunity comes. . . .

However, it must be remembered that the mental capacity of about 60% of the patients is in such a low state that they can never be self-supporting and are at a loss when left to their own resources, hence the necessity of establishing institutions for their maintenance and care.

Kupelian also mentioned that Pownal's employees had been organized into a permanent fire fighting force, a fact that readers might come to appreciate later when they learned of major blazes at the school. All ward buildings were provided with chemical fire extinguishers and fire escapes; in addition, ladders, hoses, and hydrants were regularly inspected.

The report closed with a somewhat gratuitous paragraph about preventing feeblemindedness:

"How was the food at Pineland?"
"Steamed."

—*Conversation with Edward B., who was placed at the Pownal State School in 1937, after being falsely accused of theft. He stayed for twenty-six years and shared his memory of them in November 2000*

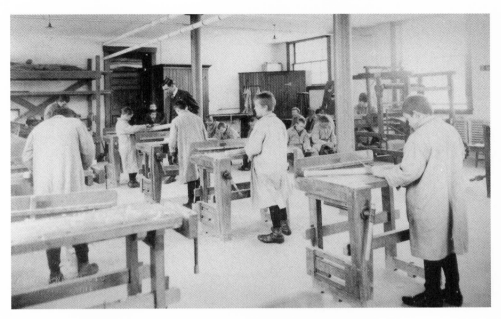

Industrial training class (courtesy of the New Gloucester Historical Society)

> *The marriage of feeble-minded in the State of Maine is prohibited . . .*
> *However, the element of illegitimacy greatly overshadows such control. An*
> *act was also passed in 1925 relating to the sterilization in certain cases for*
> *the prevention of the production of feeble-mindedness. . . . Since then there*
> *is the record of 72 eugenic sterilizations in Maine. Considering the fact*
> *that the sterilization law in Maine has been in effect for thirteen years, this*
> *comparatively small number of cases is disappointing, and apparently a*
> *widespread application of these operations cannot be expected.*

Bureaucratic Divorce

Kupelian's reassurances to the public failed to mention the various social and political forces then swirling around the state, including two critical to the school's immediate future. One was continuation of loud objections to the linking of health programs and criminal institutions in the government reorganization of 1932. The second was a legislative skirmish over the fate of Commissioner Leadbetter. The two came together in 1939.

A career administrator and survivor who had long operated at the center of state power and served the state's governor and council as messenger, Leadbetter was now the target of legislators seeking to "tighten up" state expenditures on

A very fine turkey dinner was served the employees on Christmas Day and the children had an especially good chicken dinner. The menus were as follows:

Employees
Fruit cup - Roast turkey
Dressing & gravy
White & sweet potato
Squash - onions
Bread - butter
Cranberry jelly
Celery - olives - pickles
Mince pie
Mixed nuts, candy & fruit
Coffee, tea or milk

Children
Roast chicken
Dressing - gravy
Squash - cranberry sauce
Bread - butter
Cracker jack - candy
Apples - oranges
Milk
Cracker jack

—*Dr. N. S. Kupelian, monthly report, December 31, 1941*

health and welfare. When the lawmakers proposed dividing the department into two parts, Governor Barrows concurred but stated emphatically that "whatever plans may be adopted . . . there will be no personal sacrifice to Mr. Leadbetter and neither will the State lose, in any degree, the benefit of his years of conscientious service and experience gained as a result." The compromise was division of the department into two pieces, with Health and Welfare continuing to administer a number of social programs and a new Department of Institutions getting Leadbetter as its leader. When the change took effect in December, he became commissioner of institutional services responsible for thirteen facilities, including the Pownal school, mental hospitals, prisons, reformatories, and sanatoriums.

The change did not happen fast enough for some legislators. In 1941, Sam E. Conner, a writer for the *Lewiston Evening Journal*, remembered that "the group behind the move was constantly kicking and cussing because the governor had not made the change the day the new law became operative." Angry legislators were already trying to oust Leadbetter again, this time by recombining the two departments. But that movement failed, and Leadbetter held on for two more years, when he retired at the mandatory age of seventy. Governor Sumner Sewall then named Harrison C. Greenleaf, a former Lewiston newspaperman, as commissioner.

> During the year several classes were held each week for both boys and girls in which they were taught to sing church music as well as songs of various types. They were taught the value of the different notes, also to write music in three keys in shapes and four-four time.
> —*Education department annual report, June 30, 1947*

The War Years

Greenleaf and Kupelian would be the two men most responsible for the Pownal school through the 1940s, and the job they faced was a big one.

Despite staffing problems, Pownal State School continued many of its earlier programs during the decade, as the director of education noted in the annual report for the year ending June 30, 1942:

> *Next year we are introducing a course in history in the 4th and 5th grades ... and I am assured that it will be a great advantage with our children. . . . The usual number of school entertainments (three) were held with the same gratifying results as in past years. . . . The Home Economics Division opened February 10th with our new dietitian as teacher. . . . Our Boy Scout Troop still maintains the high standard for scouting activities as in the past. . . . Three of our Camp Fire Girls attended Camp Hitinowa at Litchfield, Maine, for the summer, earning their way by washing dishes and doing kitchen work. . . . In October the Camp Fire Girls, assisted by the Bluebirds and Beavers, presented a musical comedy, "King Melody's Musical Festival." . . . In April, Miss Blake, the guardian, received the medal for the most outstanding work in Camp Fire. . . . She also received the WAKEN honor which is the highest National honor to be awarded.*

School activities did occasionally change to help meet war needs. Pownal's Boy Scouts, said the same report, had collected 720 pounds of rubber as well as metal, grease, and fats from local homes, in addition to more material from the school itself. The school's troop was, in fact, the only one in the area known to be collecting grease and fats.

Celebrations continued, too. Fourth of July activities included flag raisings, "horribles parades," field shows, and stunts. Christmas included special meals and the distribution of gifts, some purchased by the superintendent and his wife on shopping trips to Portland and some contributed by the community outside the school. A 1945 report listed packages and cards received, inspected, and distributed by Pownal officials:

> The serious shortage of registered nurses continues. Before the war we had approximately fourteen and at present we have only four. The lack of trained nurses has greatly curtailed the activities of hospital wards. As the result, we were forced to teach as much as possible to the new employees and higher grade boys and girls in the care of sick children. However, every effort was made to keep the hospital standard as high as possible.
>
> —Dr. N. S. Kupelian, annual report, June 30, 1947

> *Incoming packages for boys and girls average about 150 packages per month; they are opened, listed, and then wrapped. At Christmas Time, since there are anywhere from 2 to 15 packages in a large box, it is quite safe to say that nearly 5,000 packages were opened, listed, wrapped and sent to the buildings for the Christmas Tree. This was done with the aid of the office girls in Medical Records, Financial and Telephone offices. In addition, packages from patients to relatives were sent out by this department. About 3,000 Christmas cards are censored during December.*

But there were troubling developments, too. Predictably, the war pulled staff from the school, and in the 1940–41 report year, employee turnover increased from 27.2 percent to 41.8 percent. At the end of the 1944–45 year, the education department would report:

> *Due to the shortage of teachers, we were compelled to combine all of the girls in our academic classes, under one teacher, and all of the boys under another, as a temporary measure.*
>
> *That same year, the boys' school closed from January on after a new teacher quit.*
>
> *He was a graduate of Colby College, interested in teaching, but with no experience. At first his discipline was fair and as his interests lay in Arithmetic, he taught this subject with a reasonable measure of success. The other subjects were more or less overlooked. In time his inexperience and lack of discipline led to his losing control and as he realized his limitations, in January after four months of service, he resigned his position.*

Conscientious objectors were assigned to work at Pineland and other institutions during the war years, but they were not many and they were not enough. In 1946, Kupelian offered summary remarks about the period:

Every effort is made to meet the needs of those who have gained admission. The prime objective is the rehabilitation of those who are capable and the promotion of good health, happiness, and contentment, among the patients. Due to the serious shortage of employees during the war years, no noticeable progress has been made. . . .

The employee situation is still serious. Although we have been able to secure additional male employees, we have not been so successful with women help, especially attendants, nurses, and teachers.

Pressures to Expand

As always, the school's supply of beds failed to meet Maine's stated needs. Demand for admission intensified as family providers for prospective patients were called to war and to work. The superintendent reported in 1946, when the waiting list contained 513 names: "The Institution is crowded to its capacity, vacancies occurring only when we have a death, transfer, or discharge. During the war years we have discharged quite a few patients who have made sufficient progress to take their places in the community." But Kupelian's "quite a few patients" was not really very many—just twenty-three in 1943, for example, when twenty others disappeared through death and forty-three new arrivals came to claim the empty beds. There might have been more; the armed services welcomed some Pownal residents as fully capable of fighting. But school officials were not eager to lose the patients most capable of surviving outside, because those were the patients they needed most to work inside.

Given the competition for vital resources, the fact that Pownal could expand its plant at all during the war was surprising. The vocational building, later called the Berman School Annex, opened its doors to classes during the final year of the conflict. In 1943, Senator Neil Bishop went to bat for the institution and called for new growth. He had been appalled at what he found there during a series of institutional visits made in the course of his fight for more sterilization:

Proper living quarters of the medical officers is imperative. I could have secured the services of two physicians if we had had suitable quarters for them. At present we cannot provide more than two rooms at the most. If a doctor has a family, he certainly is entitled to more than two rooms. If we are to attract desirable medical men, living conditions must be attractive.

—*Dr. N. S. Kupelian, annual report, June 30, 1945*

[O]ver at Pownal, we found deplorable and horrible conditions. . . . We found one family there of six children, all in the low-grade bracket, their mother and father still at large, still reproducing and still supplying material for the institutions. We saw some of the most horrible sights that any person can imagine.

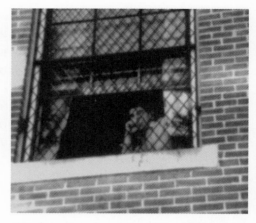

Window view (courtesy of the Maine State Archives)

Bishop chose not to renew the battle for sterilization at that point. But he did submit a bill to fund a new building to house employees. The legislature set aside $100,000 for construction when war conditions allowed, and the new twenty-eight-room building, complete with recreational, kitchen, and laundry facilities, opened in November 1946. Later known as Bishop Hall, the structure could house fifty workers and would serve well for decades before decaying to the point that its destruction would be necessary in the year 2000.

In 1944, meeting in special session, legislators approved two new dorms to house 400 more patients at the school, along with expansions of the state fish hatchery and their own salaries. As the decision approached, Sam E. Conner conveyed to readers of the *Lewiston Evening Journal* his own enthusiasm for the project:

With 1,076 patients in the Pownal home for feeble minded, their beds placed so close together, by force of necessity, that it is necessary to walk sideways to pass between them, there can be no successful argument that the institution is not over crowded.

This will, practically, clean up the waiting list and for the present at least be a stop gap in the situation. . . .

These plans and specifications will show the law makers that they are not being asked to provide money to make a handsome showing, but rather to give the home two buildings of the very latest in modern design, for such work, of simple but substantial construction. No frills, no furbelows are planned. Everything proposed is practical and for a practical purpose.

An unfortunate affair occurred during the night of October 25. It appears that one of our employees came to his room under the influence of liquor and a quarrel followed between him and his wife. While some of our boys were patrolling the grounds, they heard a woman screaming and immediately notified the night watchman who is also a deputy sheriff. It was stated by the deputy sheriff that this employee created quite a disturbance which he heard from the grounds some distance from the building. He further states he heard the employee's wife screaming and she evidently was being beaten up. Not realizing what he would be faced with he withdrew his gun and went into the room. When the employee began protesting against the admonitions he used profane language. At this moment the deputy saw the employee grasp his wife by the throat and throw her on the floor, and turned to jump on the deputy to knock him down. During the tussle, the gun exploded piercing the employee's neck. This was apparently accidental. The patient was transferred to the hospital by stretcher and an examination done by me showed that the wound was not serious. The State Police was notified. He came soon after and took statements from both parties. The wound was superficial, penetrating the left side of neck along the level of the left angle of the jaw following a course upward and backward lodging under the skin of the left occipital region. The bullet was removed under local anesthetic. The patient made a good recovery. During an interview with the Superintendent, the employee admitted his fault and under the circumstances he thought it was best for him to leave the employment.

—*Dr. N. S. Kupelian, monthly report, October 31, 1947*

There will be no wooden floors or wainscots. Floors will be tile and wainscots of the same material up for about 6 feet. Above that point walls will be of plain brick painted. . . .

The plans for these two dormitory buildings are ultra modern and in complete accordance with the latest developments in this line of building. . . .

To those unfamiliar with the developments in this work of caring for the feeble minded the most drastic change will be the total absence of corridors. Each building will have four wings, each of which will be one complete room with a capacity of 50 patients, instead of, as was the old practice, being divided into four rooms by corridors dividing the building in the centers. . . . These dormitory rooms will open into another large room

HELP WANTED

The Pownal State School at Pownal now has openings in the following positions for persons qualified for employment and interested in steady work in State institutions. A PERMANENT JOB COUNTS NOW.

All applicants, in order to receive consideration, must be of good character and able to furnish references. Honorably discharged veterans of World War Two will receive preference.

MALE AND FEMALE ATTENDANTS

DIETITIAN   REGISTERED NURSES   COOKS

These positions offer you permanent employment. Each carries cash salary and full maintenance, including board and room. Pleasant working conditions; regular paid vacations and holidays; sick leave and state pension rights.

Please apply in person or in writing to N. S. KUPELIAN, M.D., SUPERINTENDENT, POWNAL STATE SCHOOL, POWNAL, MAINE.

Signed: HARRISON C. GREENLEAF

Commissioner

Dept. Of Institutional Service

—Text of a postwar ad that appeared in various newspapers

which will provide an assembly and recreation room for cold weather and stormy days, when such inmates as are able to do so cannot get out of doors. . . .

Construction of the two buildings, which would house patients with severe retardation and be known as Bliss Hall and Kupelian Hall, was delayed until after the war and did not end until 1949. The cost was double what had been anticipated, and the first new structure sat empty for a time until additional funds could be found for furnishings. With both buildings completed and outfitted, Pownal State School reached a residential capacity of 1,500.

Fires and Escapes

Before the new buildings were even started, some old ones had disappeared. Kupelian told the story succinctly in his monthly report for April 1945:

On April 2, Jean Gamache escaped at 4 A. M. He set fire to four barns, two of which burned flat. They were known as the Goff and Middle barns. Jean was apprehended by the Waterville police and returned by Dr. Kupelian. He was then placed in the Cumberland County Jail by Deputy Sheriff Durgin of Gray. On April 3, Dr. Kupelian brought charges against Jean in the Portland Municipal Court. He was held on $10,000 bail and returned to the Cumberland County Jail to await action of the Grand Jury which will meet in May.

Gamache, it turned out, had been sentenced to prison the previous year with an order that he be transferred immediately to Pownal. He had pleaded guilty to setting three fires in Brunswick and was suspected of setting four more. "I am convinced that the boy should not be punished in a penitentiary but should be confined and treated at Pownal school for the feeble-minded," his judge concluded. Gamache escaped briefly from the school in November and December 1944; he had placed a dummy in his bed before leaving for his April adventures, which eventually took him back to state prison.

A few months later, another inmate burned another barn. "He made such contradictory statements," Kupelian reported, that "we could not state definitely why he burned the barn. However, it must be remembered that Jean Gamache left our boys with the idea that if they wanted to get out of this institution they could do so by burning buildings."

Fortunately, most residents tried other approaches to leaving. Some went home on short visits and leaves, after their families had made formal requests to have them. School administrators of the period received thirty or so requests a month for such visits, and they often approved about half. Reasons offered for refusal included "erotic tendencies" of the patient and frequent use of alcohol at home.

Others inmates, like many before them, simply left the grounds without notice. A common route away from the grounds was along the Maine Central Railroad tracks that ran nearby; people who lived along the route would sometimes look the other way or even lend a hand, as did the farmer who owned the barn where Charles O. Wyman spent a night in 1927. Most escapees were found quickly and

---

On August 15, 1945, the full [Boy Scout] troop hiked to Freeport, Maine, where they participated in the Victory Parade, helped to build a Council Fire Ring in the town park, and assisted in recovering the body of a person drowned in the swimming pool.

—*Dr. N. S. Kupelian, annual report, June 30, 1945*

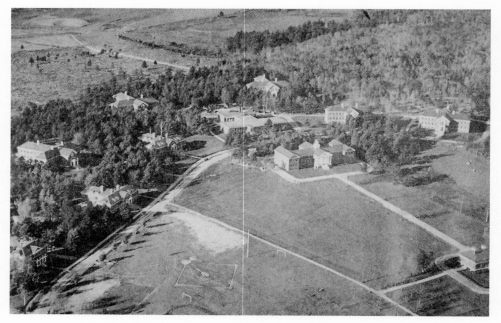

Aerial view of Pownal State School (courtesy of the New Gloucester Historical Society)

returned to the school, but a few, such as Wyman, stayed away long enough for authorities to scratch them off the books and forget them, thus freeing a bed to be filled by somebody else. Escapes were common enough for the school to create a notebook to list them. The small leatherlike notebook had ESCAPE BOOK printed in gold-colored ink on the cover. Whoever designed the volume was thinking big. It had 292 pages, each with thirty lines and printed column headings. The first entry is for September 30, 1946, and the last for May 26, 1977. There were thirty-five escapes in 1947 and forty in 1951, but many fewer in later years (one in 1975, three in 1976). Most of the book's pages were empty when it landed in the state archives after the school closed.

A definite policy has been decided upon for the payment of wages to our girls placed out for domestic service. Beginning the week of November 11, one week the money will be paid personally to the girl, and the alternate week it should be sent to Pownal State School to be deposited for the girl.
—*Dr. N. S. Kupelian, monthly report, November 30, 1940*

Postwar Problems

Some of the problems faced by the Pownal school in the postwar years, such as escape attempts, were typical of similar schools, and some were typical of almost any residential institution housing more than a thousand people. There were medical emergencies and accidents, and disputes among employees. There were deaths of patients confined for life. There were troubles with crops caused by weather and pests. There were out-of-tune pianos, and snowstorms that kept movies from arriving on time. There were roads with potholes, machines that failed, and, at one point, some unwanted cats reproducing beneath one of the buildings, a fact duly reported by Kupelian to the commissioner in Augusta.

Other problems were products of the postwar economy. Meat was hard to get at one point, flour at another. Lumber was tough to find, too, and it was badly needed. "There are about 60 buildings within the Institution," Kupelian said in June 1946. "It is no small task to keep them in good repair." The school had purchased a secondhand sawmill the previous year, he said, and had already cut 70,000 board feet of lumber for its use.

At the end of the next fiscal year, in June 1947, Kupelian summarized a few more difficulties:

> The administrative problems of the fiscal year just ended have been most difficult to cope with successfully. Since the cessation of World War II hostilities, our inability to match the lucrative salaries offered by outside industry has created a shortage of skilled labor within the institution. It has been more difficult to supply adequate food for children and employees than it was during the war years. The skyrocketing of prices on all commodities was beyond our control when the budget was prepared two years ago, thus creating a deficit in our appropriation.

The following year the school created the post of business agent to help contend with some of the difficulties. The job went to Edward P. Witham, Jr., who would stay until 1967 and make enough impact to have a small pond on the grounds—previously known as "the frog pond"—named after him.

Postwar problems also reflected a changing patient population at Pownal. New drugs and medical procedures were preserving lives that once would have ended

It is prohibited for employees to read children's letters. They are censored in the Office, which is sufficient.

—*Dr. N. S. Kupelian, notice, January 28, 1944*

I enjoyed so much our meeting at Pownal and wish I might go again and see all the buildings. Anyhow I saw the need of much our citizens could do if they knew and wished.

I have done a little missionary work for you. Last Thursday I took the matter up at Opportunity Circle of the Cong. Church here of which I am Vice. Pres. I asked for a dime for clothing and twenty-five dollars to buy cotton cloth for girls dresses. They gave me the money and told me to buy it. Am I right in thinking they need cotton cloth for dresses? Is that the most needed? I saw how cleverly they were mending up clothes in the mending room.

—Mrs. Charles M. Hobbs of Farmington to Dr. N. S.
Kupelian, after a visit to Pownal in 1947

The dress material that you sent to the girls is very pretty and you have used excellent taste in choosing it. . . .

It is unfortunate that the citizens of Maine know very little about the Institutions of the State. If they would visit them more often and see the conditions with their own eyes, I am sure our work would be much easier than it is now. After all, the Legislature will expend money when there is a demand from the citizens of Maine. I feel that citizens should know more not only about Pownal State School but about other State Institutions. These Institutions are supported by their tax money, and they should visit them to see how that money is spent.

—Dr. N. S. Kupelian, responding to Mrs. Hobbs, May 5, 1947

earlier. The courts were directing delinquents to the school, thanks to legislative action in 1941, and at least one court demanded that the school open more spaces to young troublemakers. In May 1946, Judge Adrian A. Cote of Lewiston refused to convict a youth for vagrancy. The boy was sick and belonged in the Pownal school, not jail, said the judge, and the fact that the school had no room for him was its fault. "Pownal authorities will leave a poor miserable soul wandering about the streets to fall into the hands of the law as a vagrant but still they keep less serious mental cases just as long as those individuals are able to do some work for them," said the judge.

Kupelian, on the other hand, was clearly worried about the low abilities of many new arrivals and the delinquency of others, as he wrote in an annual report produced in June 1947:

Of all admissions during the period of September 25, 1946 to November 8, 1947 almost 39% have an I.Q. below 30, requiring infant care such as dressing, bathing, toilet care, feeding and bed care. Some are unable to speak, sit up, or turn over, several are epileptics or have some kind of epileptiform convulsions. . . . Of all admitted during this period one girl, a transfer from Skowhegan Reformatory, and four boys seem physically and mentally promising to be trained to be useful in institution or later return to society. This ratio of admission is incompatible with the original purpose of the school, which is not to be an infirmary for the physically and mentally helpless and a convenient dumping ground for the troublesome but an institution for training the somewhat mentally handicapped to return to community life. Meanwhile bed patients, epileptics and ambulatory idiots and low grade imbeciles must be cared for, and with the decrease in high grade patients more of the work will have to be done by attendants, calling for an increased personnel and increase in appropriation.

In 1941 the 90th Legislature passed the so-called "Juvenile Defective Deficiency Act" authorizing the Municipal Judges to commit to Pownal State School juvenile defective delinquents. These cases have created a serious administrative problem . . . .

Still another set of postwar problems appeared to signal, if very faintly, new general attitudes and concern about institutions for the retarded. Across the nation, conscientious objectors who had spent some of their war years in schools such as Pineland were exposing the difficult conditions they had found, the sad and frightening results of the Depression and the war, and public inattention. In Maine, a similar job was taken on by the Maine Federation of Women's Clubs. In 1946, the federation told Governor Horace A. Hildreth of its concerns about Maine's mental institutions. The governor responded by asking the federation to investigate conditions at the Augusta State Hospital, the Bangor State Hospital, and Pownal State School. The resulting report made the headlines on February 6, 1947, and served notice that all was not well. The three institutions were terribly crowded, it

---

It has been a tremendous task during the war years to carry on the institutional activities efficiently. This has been possible by self-sacrifice and devotion of the older employees and their willingness to serve for the best interest of the Institution.

—Dr. N. S. Kupelian, annual report, June 30, 1946

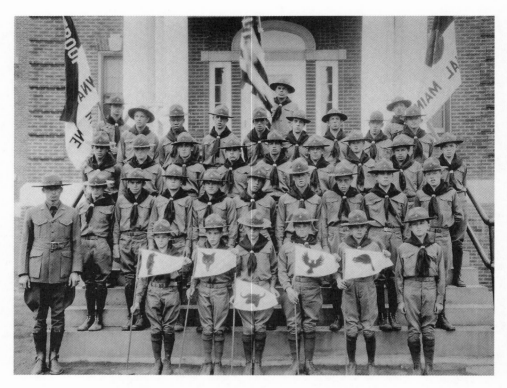

Boy Scouts on show (courtesy of the New Gloucester Historical Society)

said, and new construction was badly needed. The report helped convince legislators to provide funds for Pownal's new dormitories despite increasing costs, but the women were not done with the state's institutions.

A New Investigation

In 1950, the Maine Federation of Women's Clubs suggested to Governor Frederick G. Payne that a new hospital visitation committee be named. The governor asked that men be included in the group, then named a dozen persons. The

> The Annual Christmas Play, "The Boy Who Did Not Believe in Santa Claus," was presented by our teachers in a very colorful and instructive entertainment. The Boy, after seeing the Toys, Dolls, Soldiers, Fairies and Santa Claus in action, acknowledged his mistake.
> —*Dr. N. S. Kupelian, annual report, June 30, 1945*

committee released a devastating report on January 10, 1951. Said the *Portland Press Herald*:

> *A 12-member Mental Hospital Visitation Committee, appointees of Gov. Frederick G. Payne, charged in a report made public today that instances of cruel and abusive treatment of patients had been uncovered at the Pownal State School.*
>
> *In a blistering criticism of the institution's administration the committee said a male patient had been scalded with hot water as punishment and a young woman had been confined for weeks to a room with broken windows in winter.*
>
> *"We are distressed by conditions we have found," the committee reported to Payne.*
>
> *Norman U. Greenlaw, commissioner of institutional services, urged instances set forth in the report "do not indicate policy nor pattern of the prescribed program at the school."*
>
> *Of the abuses alleged, Greenlaw said:*
>
> *"The abuses referred to in the report appear outrageous and to some extent are as reported, but to accept them as given is neither fair nor objective."*
>
> *Dr. N. S. Kupelian, superintendent of the institution for feeble-minded, maintained many charges by the committee were false.*
>
> *"I believe the committee came to Pownal to find fault. That was their attitude from the start," said Doctor Kupelian. . . .*
>
> *The committee, in prefacing its allegation of cruel and abusive treatment, said:*
>
> *"We have been told by both present and former attendants that if you knew what goes on at Pownal, you could not sleep nights. In the light of what we stumbled onto, we cannot too much discount their statements."*

The Boy Scouts and Pioneers were active about their camp in the woods nearby. They have named it Moose Run through the fact that moose tracks are very much in evidence near the camp. The boys have moved the small building on the camp site to allow more space in the clearing, and installed new windows, new roof, and laid a new floor. They placed a barrel over the spring nearby and developed a swimming hole in the brook. The time and interest spent on this project is an asset to the physical activities of the school.

—*Education department report, June 30, 1949*

A large number of patients were confined to straitjackets, said the report, "although the use of such is rather generally regarded as a relic of the dark ages." A man who was fastened to a bed had his hands caught between the bars of the bed until they were swollen and discolored, but there were no attendants on the ward to assist him. Every building seemed "surgically clean," but there was "no evidence of rehabilitative work." Kupelian himself gave conflicting information about X-ray machines and other matters, and the staff had too few doctors and assistants. In fact the doctor and the hospital could do as much as it did only because patients had been trained to help—a fact that disturbed the investigators. "We contend," they wrote, "that any patient who has the emotional stability and intelligence to help in surgery could and should be outside Pownal."

Said one summary paragraph (without identifying the person speaking as "I"):

> *Doctor Kupelian said that on pleasant days they would be outdoors, but one wonders where they would sit for there were in that area seats for not more than 30, even though such furniture is being made in the workshop. Merely custodial care—however cleanly and sanitary—is not too great an advance from the old bedlam, and for anyone who thinks that statement extreme I recommend their spending some time in Yarmouth Hall at Pownal.*

Dr. Kupelian had devoted almost three decades of his life to Pownal State School. He had played a vital role in building its population from 300 to 1,500 patients during some of the nation's most trying times. He had tried hard to win new resources, to hire new people. He had cared and done his best, and he greeted the charges with anger.

> *This committee wanted to paint a bad picture. They never asked me what we did for betterment. They never mentioned we have motion pictures twice a week, that we have religious services every day and that frequent outside entertainment comes to us.*

> In reviewing the year it is interesting to note that the majority of subjects coming from outside for examination were brought by parents or other relatives rather than by Social Workers. Naturally, most of these parents were doubtful and troubled. Frequently much more time was given to their emotional needs and problems than was required for the examination of the subjects.
>
> *—Ernestine Porter, report of Psychological Service, June 30, 1952*

Fourth of July—Pownal

July 4—I am going to interrupt for this week my series on "Women Who Danced" to bring to my readers the experience of today at Maine's noblest institution for deserving but unfortunate children.

My admiration for Dr. Kupelian and his wife, already great, was increased greatly today. He is much more than a Superintendent, he is a splendid doctor whose heart is in his work, and his devotion to these wards exceeds the line of duty. They showed their love and their appreciation of his many kindnesses as the Girl Scouts in the Pyramid Act extending on the ground sat up and sang "Happy Birthday to you, Dr. Kupelian." His birthday is tomorrow. Then they rose, forming a living beautiful "K" in formation; then again in perfect "P" for his son in the armed service. Dr. Kupelian, much moved, thanked them from his heart.

Picture a 16-acre quadrangle between the Administration Building and the Hospital, a hot sun, great fleecy clouds floating overhead, a large crowd waiting for the start of the parade; and here it comes. Away off on the right flank were the Girl Scouts in their costumes, all with bright red stockings, then rapidly, men and women falling in from Hill Farm; Valley Farm; Hospital, Cumberland Hall, Pownal Hall, New Gloucester Hall; Gray Hall; Vosburgh Hall; Staples Hall; and Yarmouth Hall; until 500 boys and girls are in motion over the great campus, marching in precision to the great flagpole in the playground. Other features were Flag raising, Camp Fire Girls and Boy Scouts, "Star Spangled Banner," sung by school. Many times in a long life I have saluted "Old Glory," but never more reverently than today. Judge was Dr. Kupelian; Field Marshals, Mr. Whittemore and Miss Blake; starter, Dr. Sturgis; referee Dr. Leach.

Events were: Hoop rolling relay, boys and girls; junior run, boys and girls; Intermediate run, boys, Pownal Hall; girls, Vosburgh hall; flag relay, boys and girls, tilting boys; pyramids girls; pillow fight, boys; horribles parade; tug of war, men; tug of war, girls and a baseball match Reds vs Blues. Umpire was Mr. McCarthy; scorekeeper, Mr. Bradbury.

"Happy Birthday, Dr. Kupelian." Thanks for the hospitality shown by you and Mrs. Kupelian to myself. Thanks to Dr. and Mrs. Leach for their gracious invitation to attend. Our appreciation to Dr. Sturgis and Alice, friend of my boyhood. God Bless Pownal, and those under the watchful care of the Loving God, always.

> —*Rev. Howard O. Hough, DD, founder and pastor*
> *emeritus, First Radio Parish Church of America,*
> *and executive director, Friendship, writing in the*
> Rockland Courier-Gazette, *July 7, 1944.*
> *Punctuation and capitalization as in original.*

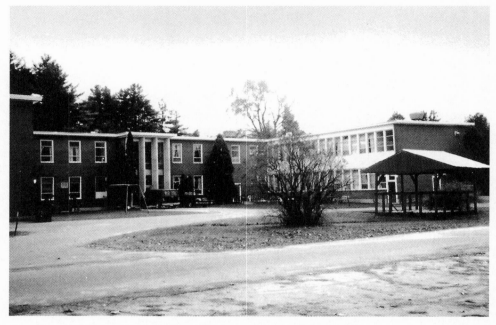

Kupelian Hall (courtesy of the New Gloucester Historical Society)

Some of the group's statements were "absolutely false," he said. Straitjackets were required for patients who abused themselves or others. As for having too few doctors and getting new ones: "I'll be very happy to have them if the committee will find them. We can't." The burns of the scalding victim were not serious, Kupelian added; he recovered in nine days.

Greenlaw supported the doctor. The attendant responsible for the scalding had been dismissed, he noted. "In its entire concept the report is unfairly misleading and points out shocking incidents and deficiencies in the program as though they portrayed the general policy rather than the exceptions."

The *Press Herald* for the following day reported that some legislators "felt they had only themselves to blame for conditions uncovered at Pownal," and that salaries should be increased. But nothing the legislature would do in the next few years would eliminate concern about the school. The new world had just collided with the old, smashing open a hole through which people could look. The citizens of Maine had just started to understand that their state was warehousing human beings in Pownal. The period of public exposé had begun.

Another Burning Barn

Attempts to raise salaries did little to pacify Pineland's employees. Staff turnover was 52.7 percent during the year that ended in June 1952 and 47.5 percent the year after that. At the end of that second year, 1,449 patients were cared for by a staff that averaged 221. The budget was increasing, but so was the number of patient applicants on the waiting list.

As always, some patients were willing to make room for others by leaving on their own volition, and in February 1953 four escaped and set fire to one of the school's large dairy barns. Staff and patients worked together in relays leading 103 cows and 3 bulls from the flaming structure, and the four escapees were apprehended the next day. But the $8,000 barn was gone, turned to ash in the final flare-up of Kupelian's career.

Now sixty-six years old, and the only fully licensed physician in an institution for 1,500 patients, Kupelian announced that he would retire on May 1. Many people would miss him; they respected him greatly, some would say later, for taking care to remember the names and observe the birthdays of residents, and for ending such disciplinary practices as shaving the heads of female residents caught talking with males. Kupelian died a few months after leaving his position, before he and his wife could begin the new life they had planned.

The name of the man who would lead Pownal State School into the second half of its life was announced in April. He was Dr. Peter W. Bowman, a resident of Medfield, Massachusetts, and a native of Hannover, West Germany. Bowman would become as solid a symbol of the new institutional age as Vosburgh and Kupelian were of the old.

All of us older employees, I am sure, feel very deeply the passing of our very good friend and superintendent, Dr. Nessib Kupelian.

In life he gave of himself until there just wasn't any more left to give. Even though he couldn't enjoy his retirement as far as worldly things were concerned, he is now living in perfect rest and peace.

His reward shall be great for having given his very best for the benefit of the sick and the unfortunate. Because of him many lives have known sunshine instead of the valley of shadows.

—Pownal Observer, *October 1953*

Part Two

Protecting People Inside by Putting Them Outside

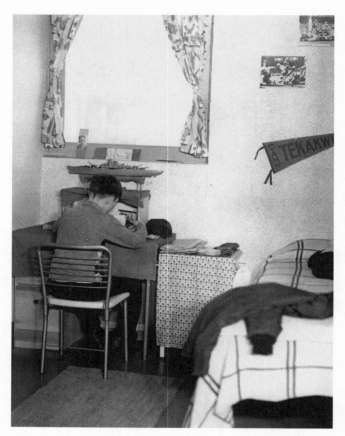

A patient at his studies (courtesy of the Maine State Archives)

The Bowman Years: 1953–1972 4

*If one is going to change things, one has to make a
fuss and catch the eye of the world.*
—Elizabeth Janeway

Dr. Kupelian was gone from the scene, but his son was not. Phillip N. Kupelian had worked at the school occasionally as a teen, driving the store truck and doing other chores. Now, having studied engineering at Boston's Wentworth Institute of Technology, he was back at Pownal State School, well into a twenty-five-year stint on the engineering staff.

Years later, Kupelian would remember some discontent and sniping among employees but an overall wonderful work experience. The place was really self-contained, he said, even though better roads had partially opened it to the larger world since his boyhood. It had everything—its own power, a blacksmith shop, a "frog pond where the kids cut ice in the winter," fireworks that he helped shoot off in July, masons and carpenters, a tin shop, steam turbines, piggeries, and hospital equipment. "I got experience in all sorts of things there. I couldn't have gotten it all anywhere else. As an engineer I couldn't have asked for more."

The first ground observation post in the United States to be built and manned by several communities was officially opened here today at the Pownal State School.

The post, built 480 feet above sea level on the roof of the school's reservoir, was named the Five Towns Post. It will serve the towns of Cumberland, Gray, New Gloucester, North Yarmouth and Pownal.

—Pownal Observer, *June 1953*

Kupelian wasn't pleased in 1958 when the school gave up generating its own electricity and purchased commercial power instead. "That sort of shot the whole business all to pieces," he said. "It ruined the self-reliant town feeling you got when you were there."

The physical plant would change a great deal in the 1950s and 1960s. But the plant, at least, was anchored in the ground. Almost everything else about the place would change even faster as new ideas swept into Maine from around the land and joined with the powerful energy of the school's new superintendent.

Forces of Change

America in the 1950s was profoundly revamping its attitudes toward retardation. Postwar exposés, some of them inspired by reports from conscientious objectors who worked in schools such as Pownal, had raised public concern about the care and non-care at such large institutions. Responses to them were often phrased in a new vocabulary. "Patients" increasingly replaced "inmates," and patients were there for their own good, not for the protection of the general public. Words such as "idiot," "imbecile," and "moron" were out. As described in literature from the Maine school, the retarded were instead divided into these three basic groups:

> 1. *The EDUCABLE, who are slow learners with an I.Q. of 50 to 70.*
> 2. *The TRAINABLE, with an I.Q. of 25 to 50 who are not capable of benefitting from usual schooling and can attain a substantial degree of limited independence and may even subsequently become gainfully employed.*
> 3. *The DEPENDENT, with an I.Q. of 25 or below who need continual supervision and care, often for such basic needs as feeding and dressing.*

If softer language helped increase people's comfort with the idea of retardation, so did admired public figures such as Pearl Buck, Roy Rogers, and Dale Evans Rogers, who revealed personal experiences with their own retarded children. Americans suddenly heard that having a retarded child was nothing to be ashamed of and that heredity played only a small part. They began to perceive that many public institutions for the retarded had so far served mostly the poor. People such as the Kennedys, who in 1962 disclosed the secret of their own retarded family member, had relied on private institutions.

We have twin kid goats at the Hill Farm barn. Goat's milk can be had by those who wish to come up and milk the goat.

—Pownal Observer, *April 1954*

> "You feel depressed at first," says a young man who has worked in the men
> and boys ward for nearly ten years. "Then you realize that they need some-
> body to care and you're stuck."
>
> —*Hazel Loveitt in* Maine Sunday Telegram,
> *September 10, 1967*

Now "well-off parents were confessing to the institutionalization of their children," according to James W. Trent, Jr., in *Inventing the Feeble Mind.* "There should
be no shame in placing a retarded child in a public facility, parents were telling each
other." So they did, and as they did, they organized to help advance the interests
of their children and to ensure their proper treatment. Numerous local and state
parental groups appeared, and in 1950 the National Association for Retarded
Children formed, soon to be assisted with financial help from Dale Evans Rogers.

As pressure for change began to mount, newspapers around the country
appeared eager to expose the faults of existing institutions. Employees desperate
for improvements sometimes assisted in the effort; in Maine, Pownal's new superintendent began sounding alarms even before the reporters did.

Dr. Peter Bowman

"The Executive council today approved the appointment of Dr. Peter W.
Bowman of Medfield, Mass., as superintendent of the Pownal State School for the
mentally deficient," said news reports of April 9, 1953. "Dr. Bowman, 33, is a native
of Hannover, West Germany, and received his M.D. degree at Goettingen, Germany,
in 1948. He and his family came to this country in 1949."

> In the face of vast appropriations of billions and billions of tax dollars
> for military purposes and for aid to other populations than our own, of
> spending billions of dollars for high-powered luxury automobiles which have
> to be kept under constant speed control by an ever-growing number of traf-
> fic police (traffic death toll 1955 approximately 37,800) it would be hypocrisy
> to refuse our mentally ill and mentally retarded citizens the humane care and
> the competent treatment which we could provide if given the tools and
> facilities.
>
> —*Dr. Peter W. Bowman, annual report, June 30, 1956*

Bowman would prove an unlikely find for the Maine school in the country. "He was brilliant," said Rose P. Ricker, a longtime coworker. "He was terrific. He had an international reputation and he had many ideas ahead of their time—like the idea that the retarded should not be isolated in places like ours. They should work and live in the community when they could."

Bowman's arrival began a movement toward professionalism in Pownal. He would build a large medical team and support further education and training for workers at every level of his staff. He would write significant medical and philosophic papers of his own, and encourage numerous research efforts by other members of his team.

"He really was way, way ahead of his time," recalled Agisilaos J. Pappanikou, Ph.D., in the year 2001. Pappanikou joined Bowman's staff as an educator in 1953. He later became a highly respected director of paramedical services, a post he held until 1965, when he moved on to the staff of the University of Connecticut, convinced that he had accomplished all he could in Maine with the resources available.

"Peter had an empathy for the downtrodden," said Pappanikou. "I think it came from what he saw in Germany during the war era. Then he came to this place that deprived people of the right to do things and he wanted to change it. So we did."

What Bowman expected when he came to the Pownal school is not in the official record, but some of what he found is included in the annual report covering his first year there:

> The fiscal year 1953/54 confronted us with unusual difficulties in providing and maintaining the most vital services at this Institution. An excessively low quota for employees in nearly all categories with a constant increase in patient population and low salaries, repetition of arson on institutional grounds, numerous attempts at derailing trains on the tracks of the Canadian National Railroad, our failure to secure a capable and competent Chief Engineer for the complicated plant operations, numerous breakdowns of equipment, prolonged illness and absence of our Food Service Manager, an epidemic of infectious hepatitis, have heavily taxed the emotional and physical resources of the executive, professional and subprofessional staffs. Periodically, unfavorable publicity in newspapers, radio, and television stations was the symptomatic confirmation of these conditions. . . .
>
> There is growing evidence . . . that we are facing unsurmountable difficulties. Common knowledge and statistics show that there is a steady increase in patient population.

The 1957 annual report included a full-page list of activity performed by the roentgenology department. It listed 3,022 X-rays—3,021 of them focused on thirty-five carefully cataloged parts of the human body. The final X-ray on the list is identified without a word of further explanation as "Examination of White Rabbit."

Even before making that report, Bowman had fed some alarming statistics to newspapers. The *Portland Sunday Telegram* reported some of them in an article by Spencer W. Campbell that ran on July 19, 1953:

> *In 1936 there were four physicians for 800 patients. Now there are three doctors for 1,480 patients. There were 14 nurses; there are six now. There was one psychologist in '36; there's one now. There are 14 teachers for the pathetically handicapped patients; there were 12 in the days when the patient load was only half as large as it is now.*

But the *Telegram* report put great hope in the school's new administrator, who had already started granting patients new freedom:

> *For the first time in nearly half a century they may smoke. And they may sample other new little pleasures that are part of normal living on the "outside."*
>
> *Such changes came to Pownal this Spring with the new superintendent, Dr. Peter Bowman, a warm, youthful, human sort of administrator who likes to remember that he's not just running an institution; he's running the lives of 1,500 patients. With him people come first.*

Bowman was not as well loved by all members of his staff. "I always thought he was a martinet," one office worker remembered years later. Others tightened up whenever he entered their labs or kitchens, their offices or training centers, for he was "quick to let you know if something was wrong."

Betty True, a kitchen worker, later remembered that Bowman "would come in and notice things and if he saw something he didn't like he would say so. Once he said the lettuce was cut too big, and the lettuce got smaller." Rose Ricker recalled the day that Bowman found staff members playing bridge in the library on their lunch break. He returned to his office to write a memo forbidding interdepartmental fraternization at lunch breaks. "I was sort of scared of him," she said. "But I admired him. He was sort of a dictator. You did things his way or you didn't do them."

People say, "take night duty at the Hospital; quiet, nothing to do," Oh Brother! You're at the desk writing in your night book, all of a sudden, Wow! What's that, a Siren? No, its just P.C., she wants to be turned over. You get pretty near back to your desk, when you wonder what's broke loose now. It's only E. H. in one of her spells. She wants a drink or wants to walk the corridors with you for company. Well you convince her she has to stay in bed.

Now you think, says I, it's quiet now, I'll start my supper. As your coffee, etc. is ready to eat, you hear a commotion up in Ward C., go on up and see M. A. in one of her convulsions or else J. K. laughing and talking to herself. Come back and record the convulsion.

Ward D. is going again, C. R. wants some warm milk, that's done, M.R. wants to be turned over and changed as she lets you know in noises of her own. Change four or five more children, and get them settled down.

Back to your coffee which by now, needs warming up, at least one bite and one swallow, the phone rings. . . .

—Pownal Observer, *April 1955*

Bowman's ability to find and report fault would be part of his eventual downfall, but for the moment it served him well as he fought for long-range change in the middle of immediate crises. There were plenty of those, as the doctor's annual report for 1955 attested. Two hurricanes had struck and paralyzed the school for days. Infectious hepatitis had broken out again. The school's much-respected, long-term director of education and Boy Scout leader had gone to prison after pleading guilty to taking sexual liberties with patients over many years. In fact, the report concluded, "1954-55 was, in all probability, the most trying of 47 years in the history of Pownal State School not only for the Staff of the Institution, but also for the Legislative and administrative branches of the State government, and for the parents of our patients."

Harry W., one of our boys, was shoveling snow at our water pumping station and as he shoveled a path to some barrels that are kept down there, a skunk emerged from under the barrels. Harry came out second best. The skunk ambled off to the woods. Harry had to stay outside the rest of the day.

—*Power Plant News*, Pownal Observer, *April 1956*

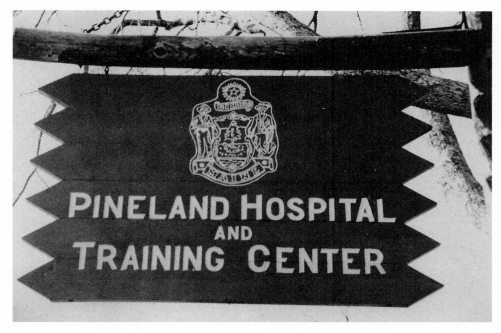

The new Pineland name (courtesy of the New Gloucester Historical Society)

Staff and Finances

Bowman would accomplish much in the 1950s and 1960s, but solving the chronic problems of staffing and funding would never make the list. In February 1954, the state released information on the sums spent daily to care for a patient

When I opened the door [of Kupelian Hall], I was shocked, it was like seeing a horror show. After a while you begin to see them as individuals, human beings needing attention. . . . Staff weren't prepared or trained to deal with various behaviors. It was hard. We did not know how. All this reflects back on the inadequacy of training. I was never prepared to see so many men naked. . . . When I walk around Pineland today, it's like "we had quite a job here." But it had such a stigma. If people could realize how much was good. The community always gets negativity.

—*Olive Church, remembering her days as a psychiatric aide to the profoundly retarded in the 1960s, as reported by Ellie Fellers in the* Lewiston Sun Journal, *May 29, 2000*

"Apples," the pet cat of the children at Staples Hall, Pineland, found a baby rabbit in the woods nearby and adopted it into her family of kittens.
—Pineland Observer, *May 1967*

in a state institution. The cost for those in general hospitals was about $10. At Bangor State Hospital the figure was $2.65. At Augusta State Hospital it was $2.28. At Pownal it was $1.98. Perhaps such information helped convince eighty-five people to meet at the school on April 4 of that year and form Pownal Parents and Friends, Associates, a group to be led in its first years by its newly elected president, Edward J. Berman, an attorney from Portland.

In 1954, Bowman testified to a legislative committee about staff difficulties. He revealed that he had fired some employees for beating and making sexual advances toward patients. He said that patients had sometimes been burned in showers because staff shortages meant they had to help one another in bathing. In all, he declared, the school required 156 new employees together with additional funds and capital construction.

Berman reinforced the superintendent's case and suggested legislative fault by adding: "Ninety per cent of the things Dr. Bowman told you are needed at this institution were publicly and repeatedly told your predecessors for the last 15 years."

A surprising if unknown number of dedicated employees stayed on at the school for years, even decades, doing their best in every way for school and patient alike. Rose Ricker was one of them. When she met Bowman in 1961, he invited her to be a "secretary's secretary," even though she then lacked a high school diploma. With his encouragement she passed an equivalency test and enrolled in courses at the University of Maine. She moved from job to job at the school, sometimes working with support staff, sometimes directly with residents, and eventually serving as librarian, chair of a research committee, and editor of the school's in-house journal, the *Observer*.

But other workers moved on. Employee turnover was 81.9 percent in 1954; a decade later, the rate in some departments was still over 60 percent.

Unions appealed to some workers, and they organized. In 1969, thirty-three members of the American Federation of State, County and Municipal Employees walked off the job for a day when a reduction in their workweek from forty-four to forty hours threatened to reduce their pay. Earlier that year, the cost of the shortened pay week (forced by a U.S. Supreme Court decision) so unnerved the *Portland Press Herald* that it suggested a study comparing state and private pay. That did not sit well with Bowman. He quickly responded with figures showing that state workers made considerably less than their privately paid counterparts. His letter to the paper, a protest that also appeared in the *Observer*, began with a strong defense of his staff:

> *Editor of the* Press Herald
>
> *After a night of wet snow and freezing rain, on Jan. 7, some 21 cars are tangled up and stalled at the foot of the hill leading to [the institution].*
>
> *These are some of the nurses, psychiatric aides, food, laundry and maintenance workers.*
>
> *They are committed and determined to report for duty to take care of their patients. Their cars could not negotiate the hill. The town plow broke down. It rests amid the bog. People try to help each other, ankle deep in snow and slush.*
>
> *That was the beginning of a working day.*

A day not made better, concluded the doctor, when the workers paused at lunch to read the *Press Herald*'s call for "some brave legislator" who would dare to reveal their pay to the public.

Bowman also took his case up the chain of command to Governor Edmund S. Muskie, offering this assessment in a memorandum prepared for a gubernatorial school visit in the spring of 1956.

> *In many buildings attendants have to handle soiling patients who are incontinent as to urine and feces. They have to handle soiled clothing, soiled linen, etc. They have to stand the smell associated with human excrement for the length of a working day. Many attendants have to handle children and adults with no appreciable power of mind. Many of these*

As in many institutions comparable to Pownal, much of the necessary nonprofessional work is carried out by the patients themselves. Without them the institution could not survive and yet in many instances their work is very much taken for granted and little appreciation shown them for what they do. Mrs. Nottage has been known, however, to turn her lakeside summer cottage over to eleven so called "working girls," with attendant supervision, so that they might enjoy a day entirely free from their duties and away from the institution. Rather than going with them herself to watch over her possessions or enjoy the outing, she stayed behind on the ward and assumed all the duties that these girls ordinarily performed.

—Pineland Observer, *May 1957*

patients have to be fed. All have to be bathed constantly and many are badly crippled and need to be carried around.

In other sections, attendants have to deal with disturbed children and also adults of higher intelligence. Their behavior might be erratic, unpredictable, sometimes threatening, and occasionally assaultive. These patients were brought here because their own parents, relatives, or social agencies were unable to handle them. The attendants are supposed to understand these patients' disturbances or if they do not understand, they still must not use physical force even though they might be alone with some 50 patients or more and they might be badly frightened. They are supposed to be emotionally mature, resourceful, and considerate.

In other words they are supposed to be good substitute parents with qualities exceeding those of parents who were unable to take care of their own children. . . .

For this type of work, the attendant is offered a starting gross salary of $42.00 per 44-hour week which is the wage for a handyman, for unskilled labor, or even less. This is certainly below the Federal minimum wage. . . .

I shall be glad to provide anyone with the opportunity of personal experience as attendant for only one day who wishes to have this experience. . . .

Profound Change

The dispute- and crisis-based headlines of the era sometimes eclipsed not only the caring and dedicated efforts of many workers to improve the lives of their patients, but also two profound changes occurring at the institution: increased emphasis on medical treatment, and a move toward deinstitutionalization. The

---

On Dec. 11, 1961, thirteen frightened and disturbed young boys and girls were admitted as patients to a new building at Pineland Hospital and Training Center. It was the beginning of a new and unusual program of psychiatric treatment for emotionally disturbed children 6-16 years old.

Only a few days earlier, Dr. Harry Solomon, Massachusetts' commissioner of mental health, said at the dedication of the Children's Psychiatric Hospital—only one in northern New England—"This is a great and daring experiment. Only time will tell how it works out."

—Pineland Observer, *March 1966*

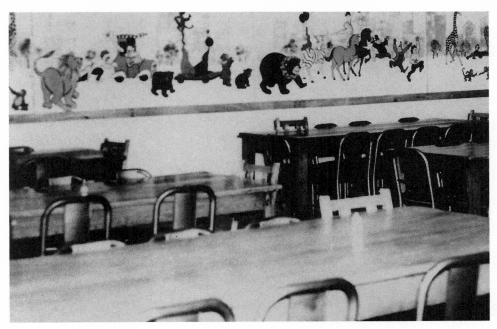

Children's dining room mural, painted by students of the Portland School of Fine and Applied Arts (courtesy of the New Gloucester Historical Society)

first of these would rename and reshape the Pownal State School; the second would eventually end its existence.

From School and Farm to Hospital

All of the school's early superintendents were medical doctors, and since 1931 Hedin Hospital had provided them space to offer more professional services to residents and some outsiders than earlier facilities had allowed. The superintendents could not give full time to medical matters, of course, because operating two farms, running school programs, and keeping residents safe from the temptations of the larger world while protecting the world from the residents occupied much of their time. But the new superintendent was not to be distracted from the medical model he envisioned as he led the school through the 1950s and 1960s.

By the end of his first year, Bowman had requested funds for a building to isolate patients with communicable diseases, hired the school's first full-time dentist, called for a competent psychiatric program, and started to search for additional medical workers.

WESTERN UNION

IT IS A PLEASURE TO SEND GREETINGS TO THE DELEGATES ATTENDING THE FIRST INTERNATIONAL MEDICAL CONFERENCE ON MENTAL RETARDATION.

BY BRINGING TO BEAR THE SCIENTIFIC KNOWLEDGE OF MANY NATIONS ON A PROBLEM WHICH KNOWS NO BOUNDARIES, THIS CONFERENCE PERFORMS TWO GREAT SERVICES FOR MANKIND: IT STRENGTHENS THE HEALTH PROGRAM OF EACH PARTICIPATING COUNTRY, AND CONTRIBUTES TO THAT SPIRIT OF UNDERSTANDING AND MUTUAL RESPECT WHICH IS ESSENTIAL TO THE BUILDING OF PEACE.

I WISH YOU WELL IN YOUR DELIBERATIONS AND ALL SUCCESS TO YOUR FUTURE WORK.

DWIGHT D. EISENHOWER

—Pineland Observer, *September 1959*

Annual reports of the institution increasingly stressed medical concerns. Summaries of surgeries performed and X-rays taken occupied more and more space, whereas reports of crops produced took less and less.

In March 1957, Governor Muskie signed a bill granting legislative approval of the school's changing purpose by giving it a new name: Pineland Hospital and Training Center. At that point Pineland already had received wide attention for its medical efforts. A national drug firm had chosen the center to research and make a movie showing the effects of a tranquilizing drug, chlorpromazine, on mentally retarded patients, and the American Psychiatric Association had given an achievement award for outstanding improvement in patient care and treatment.

Two years later, Bowman and his associates played leading roles in organizing a highly professional gathering in Portland, the First International Conference on Mental Retardation. That event brought together 500 experts from thirty-five nations, many of whom visited Pineland to examine the institution's expanding treatment programs. The conference yielded published proceedings that would circulate around the world.

More medical treatment required more medical buildings. In 1961, Pineland dedicated both the Perry D. Hayden Infirmary, for 130 patients requiring custodial care, and the Children's Psychiatric Hospital, which had 70 beds for emotionally disturbed children. Two hundred guests attended the first opening, and psychiatric experts from around the country came to the second.

Research reports from Bowman and others were becoming common, and some were published in a bulletin from the Frank D. Self Foundation, Inc., a research organization founded by Pineland Parents and Friends Associates, Inc. One of these concerned the study of chlorpromazine, which was found to improve the behavior but not—as some had reported—the intelligence of the retarded.

Tranquilizing drugs were increasingly prescribed as doctors learned more about their use and sometimes misuse. "Tranquilizers of various types were used more freely this year," Bowman reported in 1957, "and although destruction of property and assaultiveness have continued in some cases, many other cases have shown marked improvement. One patient camisoled [in a straitjacket] for years now sits quietly and without restraint but interestingly enough in a position as though still restrained."

The medical staff increased as facilities grew. The annual report for 1962–63 named an administrative staff of just six but a medical staff that included twelve medical doctors. The same report listed a consulting staff with twenty-four doctors, five psychiatric medical doctors, three psychology consultants, and a medical sociologist.

Care provided through the new medical emphasis was good enough to earn national approval. In November 1963, Pineland won full accreditation from the Joint Commission on Accreditation of Hospitals, the first such approval in the school's fifty-five-year history.

By the end of the Bowman era, Pineland was not just for the retarded, as its annual report for 1968–69 made clear. Hedin Hospital had for years offered short-term services for patients from other institutions, but the creation of the psychi-

---

Although the original building is still used, Pineland has grown into the third largest hospital in Northern New England (New Hampshire State Hospital, Augusta State Hospital, first and second) and probably the most overcrowded one in all New England. . . .

Peaceful farming for the purpose of keeping adult retardates busy (and institutionalized) has been replaced by a modern program which includes nursing care, medical care, psychiatric treatments, special education, psychodiagnostic and psychometric evaluation, speech therapy, physical therapy, music therapy, occupational therapy, recreation and a limited physical education program.

—*Dr. Peter M. Bowman, reporting in the* Pineland
Observer *of October 1959, in Pineland's fiftieth year*

> Therefore it is obvious that to provide the extras and little things that make a child's life happier, richer and fuller we must look forward to our friends to supply these items. They are badly needed and they do give this extra meaning to life to our lifelong children.
>
> *—From a manual for volunteers at Pineland*

atric hospital had made a more profound change. Bowman's position is described by the 1968–69 report as "Superintendent, Hospital for Mentally Ill." And Pineland now offered "two types of services for the people of Maine," the report said. "The first is for the training, education and treatment of the mentally retarded. A second is for the care and treatment of mentally ill children between the ages of six and sixteen."

The annual reports for the late 1960s no longer mentioned Pineland's farm operations at all. New medical programs might win research grants and federal funds, but these could not compensate for the state's tight budget. With the increased resources and attention being given to medical programs, something else had to give, and the farms were likely candidates. The Hill Farm closed in 1961. The Valley Farm would provide milk and beef to Pineland for a while longer, but the 1961–62 farm report contained bleak news of other farm operations:

> At the Piggery there have been 195 pigs born, of which 35 were sold to other institutions. 152 hogs were butchered, from which 34,514 pounds of pork were used by the institution. The average weight per hog was 227 pounds.
>
> Due to a number of factors such as labor, equipment and other facilities, it has been decided that it would be wise to discontinue the pigs and hogs.
>
> Also, it has been decided that we close our poultry plant.
>
> It was also decided to drop crops of vegetable raising.

The Valley Farm closed in 1967, but all outdoor operations did not end; the vocational education department that same year started an apple orchard with 95 trees, pruned 10,000 pine trees, maintained 300 pheasants to be released by the Maine Fish and Game Department, and stocked a fishpond with 500 trout.

From Hospital to Community

In the first year of Bowman's administration, fifty-six residents were discharged from the school. That was "the most ever for Pownal," according to a 1968 retro-

I remember a boy in the hospital. He was like nine or ten, maybe. He had shot his brother accidentally and he didn't remember it. He had killed him. His mother sent him there, and he spent a lot of time coloring pictures to give his brother. One night I heard him crying. I went in and found out the boy's memory had come back. I got the doctor and stayed with the boy. That was the hardest night I ever put in. But a month or so later he was better and he went home.

—*Wayne Haskell, a psychiatric aide in Children's Psychiatric Hospital, remembering back in the year 2000*

spective in the *Pineland Observer*. The discharges also suggested an idea that might have stunned Superintendents Vosburgh and Kupelian: that many retarded people should live not in institutions such as Pineland but in the larger community.

The concept of deinstitutionalization gained strength around the country in the 1960s. But Bowman advanced it in Maine some years before that. He may have been prompted in part by finding in the school's population some residents whose testing and records were incomplete but who seemed very capable of existing out-

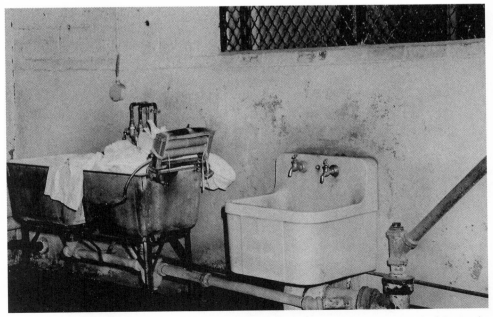

Antiquated equipment in Kupelian Hall (courtesy of the New Gloucester Historical Society)

side the facility. Bowman said in December 1953 that 300 patients had never been diagnosed at all because of staff shortages. New tests confirmed the potential of many residents. The institution's population did continue to grow through the 1950s, and there was still a waiting list, but faces as well as needs were changing.

By October 1962, according to an *Observer* report on the school's first sixty years, "the ever-present waiting list had again grown to 200 names, despite the fact that 400 patients had left Pineland over the previous three years to move into nursing or boarding homes. At Pineland there were over 300 totally dependent patients, and the number was slowly growing." A pattern first noted by Vosburgh continued: People with fewer needs were moving out, and people with more needs were moving in. But now the total population was going down. In the late 1950s the enrollment had risen to almost 1,700—although the number actually on the campus at any one time was closer to 1,500. By June 30, 1969, the number of patients present had decreased to 826; there were 75 in the Children's Psychiatric Hospital and 751 in the retarded section.

A booklet produced by the school to describe itself in the 1960s captures the spirit of the new philosophy saying on the front cover, "'The Mentally Retarded and Ill Can Return - - - Somehow - - - Somewhere - - -'"; on the back cover, "'Training and Integration' NOT 'Segregation and Detention.'"

A Defense of Change

Another booklet published by the school, "A Case for Community Placement," gives a spirited defense of the new way. Written in 1962 by John L. Hoffman, Pineland's social research scientist, the pamphlet begins with these observations:

I would greatly appreciate it if you would circulate this letter to the patients who are about to be discharged so that I might contribute a little bit to their future.

As you probably know through my records, I am an epileptic, and it was a concern to me and to my family to what was in store for me in life after my release from the hospital. Well, for the first few months it was kind of hard, but with patience and understanding, I conform, and today I know that if it hadn't been for Pineland Hospital, I might not be well off as I am today. This Hospital and Training Center is not a place of desperation but a place for the hopeless.

—*Former patient*, Pineland Observer, *January 1965*

Although we are very pleased to see our girls leave the Institution and go out to work, it leaves less hands to do the mending. We once had 14 sewing machines and one darner operating. Last month we had 3 sewing machines and the darner.

After some discussion, the only solution appeared to be hiring of employees. . . .

—Laundry department report, October 1958

Not too many years ago it was generally believed that both the State and some persons, considered to be "feeble-minded," were best served if these persons were placed in an institution, usually for the rest of their lives. . . .

Since 1953, Maine has placed increasing emphasis on the education or training of many of its retarded in Pineland to help give them some kind of life in the "outside" world rather than keeping them forever behind high custodial walls in an increasingly overcrowded institution.

This change in care and treatment, as with many other changes in society, has not yet met with entirely unanimous approval.

There are many persons in our State who still adhere to the belief in, and desirability of, strictly custodial treatment.

There are several ways of discussing certain social problems. One is on a wide statistical basis with considerable numerical data.

Another is to consider a particular case history and the effects of a particular social system upon an individual. . . .

This paper deals with an individual.

Mary Smith, as the booklet called her, had forged several checks for small amounts to buy clothing in 1919, the year her father died. She was seventeen. Sentenced to a reformatory for five years, she was tested, pronounced retarded, and transferred to Pownal State School for an indeterminate period. For years Mary's mother wrote to the school asking for her return, but the school refused time and again, and the two women could communicate only by mail. Their letters, quoted extensively by Hoffman, are heartrending. After Mary's mother died in 1941, Mary began to decline into madness. In 1952 the school transferred her to the Bangor State Hospital for the Insane.

Hoffman's summary was angry:

For a relatively minor offense, committed when she was a teen-aged girl, Mary Smith served a sentence of over 33 years of regimented and unnatural detention away from her home and family and friends, with whom she longed to be.

She was for many years described as a good and competent worker at the Pownal State School, and her intelligence tests placed her in the educable group; one test put her at the very top of this group.

The educable retarded are considered as having the greatest potentiality for normal social adjustment and employability.

Yet in all 33 years of her detention, Mary Smith was not given a single chance to try to exist in the outside world.

Not even one brief visit to her home to see her mother and relatives.

We feel a kind of collective and corporate crime was committed against this girl, which was far greater than any wrong she herself had done, or indeed was ever capable of doing. . . .

Surely this history of Mary Smith shows that an antiquated program, capable of creating this kind of misery, cannot be restored.

It tells us that we must strive, as we have in recent years, to continue and to perfect far more humane approaches and answers to the problems of mental retardation.

How much impact Hoffman's booklet had on immediate events is not clear, but movement from hospital to community continued in a wave that some would later call "the first exodus."

On occasion we have chided members of the Maine Legislature for what appeared to be failure to display the sort of political fortitude a given situation demanded.

So we are grateful for an opportunity to render solemn salute to the lawmakers for an act of raw courage which, though not unprecedented, certainly is uncommon enough to merit special recognition.

The House last week gave approval to a pay raise of $50 for members of the next legislature. . . .

Lesser men might have been deterred by the knowledge that mentally retarded young people won't be getting the care and instruction they need because salaries are so low that it is impossible to keep a professional staff at Pineland Hospital and Training Center.

—Pineland Observer, *June 1969*

> Bowman went as far as he could possibly go with what he had. . . . We built a gym and a church and a major speech and hearing center. We had the first international conference on retardation. We did things no other small institution did. . . . Pineland was an exciting place to be, a fertile place to be in those days.
>
> —*Agisilaos Pappanikou, Ph.D., January 2001*

New Buildings and Programs

In 1956, Pineland had housed 1,468 patients in dormitory space certified as adequate for 913 beds. With the number of patients dipping into the 800s and heading lower, it might seem that no new construction would be needed, but that was not the case. The more seriously retarded patients now filling many beds required different facilities, such as the new infirmary. Preparing other patients for community life required new programs, and some of these also required a new physical plant.

Efforts at academic, occupational, and physical training all intensified, with the speed dependent on the availability of funds and staff. In a first for institutions of its kind, the school established a driver training course for selected patients in 1957. The primary goal of the program was teaching highway safety, according to the *Observer*, but some graduates drove extensively after leaving Pineland.

Two years later, the department of psychology wrote of three major training needs for patients returning to the community. Sex education was one. "Ignorance in this area has added considerably to the fears, anxieties and conflicts of our most promising patients," said a department report. Promoting realistic work habits was another. "Somehow," said the report, "we must overcome the easy-going institutional pace, if these patients are to survive in the community." A change of attitude toward patients breaking rules was the third need. "Not a tightening of rules and restriction of activity, but a recognition that misbehavior offers an opportunity for teaching and explanation and is part of the learning process."

Some new programs involved outside assistance. Among the most impressive was a work training program conducted by the Hillcrest Poultry Company in Lewiston, which welcomed capable Pineland patients into its workforce for initial training and eventual full employment at union wages. "This is one of the most progressive steps we have ever been able to take in our long-range rehabilitation program at Pineland," Bowman said.

The list of plant changes during the Bowman era is impressive. In 1958 came the Benda wing of the hospital, a new school, the Federation Village apartments for employees, and a new laundry. Doris Sidwell Hall was dedicated in 1960. A "homelife cottage" for sixteen girls, it contained eight double bedrooms, four baths, a living room, dining room, and kitchen, and space for two staff members. It was based on arguments such as these from Bowman:

> Who can expect a simple mind to know the difference between mine and thine if there is only thine? How can it be expected of a girl to clean a bedroom, arrange furniture, hang curtains, vacuum a rug and use a napkin, if she has never seen bedroom furniture, curtains, rugs, vacuum cleaners, or napkins?

In 1965 the Governor Edmund S. Muskie Treatment Building joined the earlier additions to the institution's medical facilities. Two years later, work began on a gymnasium that school friends and officials had been requesting since 1912, according to the *Observer*'s calculations. A year after that, Bliss Hall reopened as a completely renovated Bliss Vocational Rehabilitation Center. Another dream became reality with the dedication of a chapel in 1970. And in 1971 workers began to renovate both Pownal and Kupelian Halls.

Outsiders at Pineland

Throughout the Bowman years, Pineland increasingly involved government and academic outsiders in its work. Some visits to the campus were carefully programmed, such as those of legislators with funding responsibilities for Pineland. "It was show and tell to keep the funding support," remembered Ellie Fellers, who worked there as a physical therapist in the early 1960s. "The word would go out that 'the legislators are coming today' and everyone would get ready to be on display."

Many other outsiders came for training; for decades, Pineland would offer formal training and courses not just to members of its own staff but to students from the University of Maine, the University of Connecticut, and other institutions.

We needed at least 300 bathing suits for patients invited to a picnic and party by a local American Legion Post. Fabian, noted TV teen-age singing idol, happened to be in town, and a station had him on a women's show (well advertised beforehand) to autograph his records free for the first 300 people who brought in new or good used bathing suits for Pineland kids. Needless to say, we had bathing suits aplenty.

—*Louis F. Moore, public education officer, 1963*

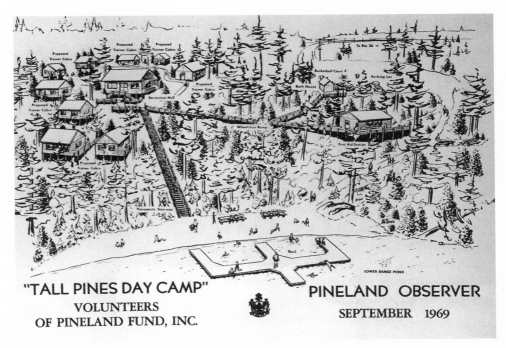

"TALL PINES DAY CAMP"
VOLUNTEERS
OF PINELAND FUND, INC.

PINELAND OBSERVER
SEPTEMBER 1969

A plan for Tall Pines (courtesy of the New Gloucester Historical Society)

"What we did was open the place," Agisilaos Pappanikou recalled. "Pineland stopped being a warehousing operation in those years. It became an open campus and we offered professional training for a lot of different people."

New Sources of Help

How could all this be? How could building and program expansion occur in the face of continuing financial and personnel problems? Bowman was still fighting these in 1969, said his annual report:

> *The fiscal year 1968/69 has been one of severe disappointments. An application for a Federal Grant to construct a pediatric service in Benda Hospital was declined because of lack of funds. Likewise, approval for a Federal Grant for our professional library was received but unfunded; therefore, no improvements could be made.*
>
> *The inflation has outpaced the cost of living increase made available to State employees with resultant poor morale and many vacancies at various levels. No meaningful new pay plan that relates to the severe loss in*

purchasing power was passed by the Legislature except in some few selected classifications.

At the beginning of the 104th Legislature, regular session, a moratorium on all new construction was proposed; thus, only funds for emergency repairs, fire safety, and remodeling of Kupelian Hall and Pownal Hall were approved.

What then were the sources of Pineland's progress? The "state legislature and governors did provide [some] money, however grudgingly," as the *Observer* stated. Staff resourcefulness also contributed to progress. When the state rejected all outside bids for a new fire station as too high, the school became its own contractor and completed the project at slightly less than what had originally been budgeted.

But the school relied for much of its growth on the fact that retardation and other disabilities were fast becoming national causes. In 1963 Congress passed the Mental Retardation Facilities and Community Mental Health Centers Construction Act. The following year came new civil rights and economic opportunity acts intended to help the disadvantaged and disenfranchised all across the land. Private foundations were also making new funds available, and Pineland was quick to benefit from them.

The Kennedy Foundation helped pay for the international conference on mental retardation held at Pineland in 1959, and Smith, Kline & French sponsored the chlorpromazine study. Federal building grants contributed to such projects as the Bliss and Pownal Hall renovations. The National Institute of Mental Health gave money for a study of brain and liver function in mental disorders. Federal sources also supported investigation of factors influencing the success or failure of patients reentering the community, a reeducation program at the psychiatric hospital, and speech and hearing labs.

We thought you'd like to know that Edward Ford and his seeing eye dog have passed the 1000 hour mark for volunteer service work at Pineland.

The courageous and generous gift of time and work by this blind man is a truly wonderful example of living a full life. How many of us could do just a little more for someone a little less well off than us?

Mr. Ford makes us see the truth of the old statement, "I cried because I had no shoes, until I met a man who had no feet."

—Pineland Progressive, *monthly bulletin of Pineland Parents and Friends, February 17, 1964*

> Tall Pines Day Camp, Poland, Maine: The opening of a day camp in June of 1969 marked the continuing investment which is being made in recreational activities for the patients at this hospital.
> Six acres of wooded land were purchased by the Volunteers of Pineland Inc. of Portland, as the first step towards the camp development.
> —*Physical Education and Recreation Report, June 30, 1969*

But there was another major force behind Pineland's growth and change—the voluntary involvement of the community beyond the grounds.

Inviting the Community In

Early school reports and literature had frequently encouraged public visits to the school, and early superintendents had bemoaned the fact that few outsiders came. But now attitudes in Maine were changing, just as they were around the country. Pownal (later Pineland) Parents and Friends Associates was one of many groups that wished to help, and the school responded with open arms to all. Soon the news of Pownal and Pineland crisis and conflict was joined in the newspapers and on the airways by a strong flow of reports describing contributions, aid, and new community connection. Society pages told of fund-raising concerts and dinners, news pages told of checks presented and purchases made, and sports pages told of Pineland soccer and other athletic teams entering contests with local schools.

A picture hung in Pineland's administration building identified Frank D. Self as the institution's first volunteer. A Second World War veteran confined to a wheelchair, he had great compassion for others and a talent for weaving that he shared with the residents of Cumberland Hall. When he died in 1953, his wife requested that friends contribute to the research fund that then bore his name.

The many new Pineland supporters who followed Self's example had remarkable energy and achieved remarkable success, so much so that other names soon joined those of the early superintendents on various buildings. The school that opened its doors in 1958, for example, became the Berman School, named for the first president of Pownal Parents and Friends. The new employee apartments were called Federation Village, to recognize the school's support from the Maine Federation of Women's Clubs. The gym became the Walter J. Soucy Gymnasium, named for a Lewiston resident who together with his wife, Louisiana, gave unmeasured time and effort to the school.

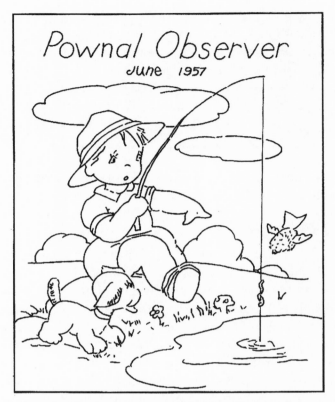

An early Observer *(courtesy of the New Gloucester
Historical Society)*

It was Soucy who headed an effort to raise funds for a new television set for
Pownal Hall in 1955. It was Soucy who sold a Lewiston carpenters' union on the
idea of building a twenty-five-passenger wooden train powered by a Jeep to carry
patients around the Pineland grounds.

"Pineland Hospital Has A Santa Named Soucy," said a headline in the *Lewiston
Sun Journal* on December 15, 1969. As usual, the article reported, the Soucys had
been collecting Christmas gifts for Pineland. Two days before, a truck from the hospital had arrived to pick up gifts, which included 1,000 pairs of shoes and boots,
1,440 candy canes, 170 toothbrushes and tubes of paste, 150 pounds of candy, 500
lollipops, 400 coloring books, 16 dozen boxes of crayons, 215 plastic model kits,
25 billfolds, 110 packs of playing cards, 117 pairs of mittens, and 5 knitted caps.

Other people were active, too, as individuals and in groups—so many that a
hundred volunteers attended the annual Volunteer Institute and Awards Program
in October 1964. In 1962, the Portland area Campfire Girls began an effort to plant

A revolutionary new program known as the "Rehab Store" started at Pineland Hospital and Training Center in Pownal in March, 1964. Thirty patients were used as a pilot group. They were given work to do and were paid for that work. With that money they could go to the Rehab Store and make their own purchases. Today more than 200 patients are involved in the "Rehabilitation Store and Work Program" as the project is known and other institutions throughout the country are asking for more information on the program and how it operates because they, too, hope to try it. . . .

Results? Astonishing. To carry money is one of the biggest privileges the children have had in the last few years. . . .

—Lewiston Journal, *February 12, 1966*

10,000 pine seedlings at the school. The next year, the Altrusa Club of Portland began seeking trading stamps in huge numbers. In May 1966, Marcel Morin of Lewiston, president of Pineland Parents and Friends, announced that the effort had netted 5.6 million stamps, enough to purchase three nine-passenger buses to help Pineland residents visit the outside world. Not long after that, the Westbrook Jaycees presented six soapbox racers to be used in Pineland's own soapbox derby.

An unusual gift came from Memorial Craftsmen of Maine, which provided headstones with names and dates to mark the graves of the 137 patients who had died and been buried in Pineland's own cemetery. The state had previously marked the graves only with numbers on small concrete posts.

One of the greatest of Pineland's many volunteer triumphs was the dedication of the All Faiths Chapel in June 1970. The $35,000 required for the building came entirely from private funds raised over fourteen years by Pineland Parents and Friends. Contributors included individuals, clubs, college groups, and churches throughout the state. "The simple and dignified wooden structure is on a landscaped plot near the administration building," said the *Maine Sunday Telegram*. "Prior to the construction of the chapel, church services for all faiths were held in the old auditorium and later in the children's dining room."

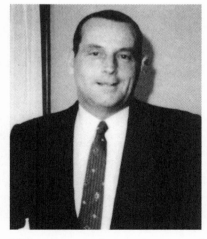

Walter Soucy, volunteer (courtesy of the Maine State Archives)

The only "crime" of these unwanted and unremembered people was that they were born mentally retarded, placed in a State institution, and then forgotten for life, by their parents, friends and relatives.

These un-named graves were for those youngsters or oldsters who, when they died, had no one to claim their body. No relative came forth or none could be found.

The only sign that they ever lived was a small piece of cement about the size of a can of tomatoes, with a number stamped on top and their names in the files of Pineland Hospital & Training Center.

Recently a large granite memorial stone with a bronze plaque, in remembrance of these un-named dead, was installed by the Pineland Parents & Friends Associates.

Since no funds were available from the State for the purchase of individual headstones for these unloved and unfortunate people they were buried in what could be termed a "Potters Field," transformed in the past ten years into a well-kept, neat and quiet small cemetery on the grounds at Pineland.

What monies could be obtained from the State Legislature for the operation of Pineland was to take care of the living, not the dead.

[Then a staff member mentioned the matter to the Memorial Craftsmen of Maine.]

The thought of these people lying in solitary loneliness in these unmarked graves bothered them too and they decided to take the solution of the problem into their own hands.

The monument makers agreed on a simple but attractive granite headstone, 18 inches high, two inches thick and eight inches wide. The full name, year of birth and year of death are stonecarved into the polished granite.

The first four of these memorials were made and put in place here Monday by Clarence Berry of the Charles A. Berry Monument Co., of Stevens Ave., Portland and the simple commemorative services were conducted by the Rev. Lee Waltz, Pineland Chaplain. . . .

These people are "forgotten" no more, thanks to determined people at Pineland and the makers of the monuments for most of Maine's cemeteries.

—Pineland Observer, *May 1964*

Successes such as this helped spur hope for more in the future. Even before the chapel opened, the Maine State Federated Labor Council spoke of adopting the children of Pineland and opened a drive to raise money for a swimming pool. The school had been trying, unsuccessfully, since 1951 to convince the legislature to fund a pool.

Volunteer services soon became so important to Pineland that the facility moved to support them with a professional effort. Mrs. Elizabeth H. Nevin became the director of volunteer services in 1960. Among her jobs was creating and maintaining a loose-leaf notebook to show to people interested in joining the effort. The introductory pages mentioned many individuals as well as fifteen groups that had helped in the past, and went on to call for more help.

> *If we could have all the volunteers we need, based on the work done by the above individuals and groups, about 50-75 a day would be required! It should be made clear that volunteers have been brought into Pineland for one reason only: To provide normal, outside contacts for our patients. In no way do they take the place of our professional staff.*

Reaching Out to the Public

Pineland's efforts to build ties with the larger community intensified again with the creation of a public relations department. Under the leadership of public information officer Louis F. Moore, the department soon took over publication of the *Observer* as well as Pineland's annual reports, then did much more, some of it indicated by Moore's annual report for 1960–61:

> *We have had many feature stories in the newspapers, giving the public a better idea of our aims and achievements, and a consequent flood of mail from the public asking for more information, or even how they might help further our program.*
>
> *We have had many spot announcements on the radio and T.V., and several ten, fifteen minute, and even half-hour shows and interviews. One*

The total valuation of Pineland Hospital and Training Center at the end of the fiscal year was $8,218,401.64. . . .

A total payroll of $3,578,096.40 was expended for the salaries of approximately 577 employees during the 1968-69 fiscal year.

The total operating cost for Pineland Hospital for the past year was $4,285,444.28

—Annual report, June 30, 1969

When the Volunteers of Pineland decided to do their May 18 Pops Concert under a tent, they went straight to a big-time tent man, Ralph Raymond of Auburn. And don't think this tent is made of anything old-fashioned like canvas, it's vinyl coated nylon, all 80 x 100 feet of it, so go to the concert, rain or shine, for the tent will be absolutely waterproof. . . .

All this we heard at the lovely dinner party which Dr. and Mrs. Peter Bowman and Dr. and Mrs. H. Jay Monroe gave at Westcustogo Inn. It was to honor, formally, the Volunteers of Pineland, and informally, several others who'd found it exciting to be of what aid they might. This struggling little band seemed not to know just what they were doing when first they organized a few years back. They didn't seem to have a great deal of support on the horizon, but each year the financial result from their Spring Ball has caused them to cry with happiness all the way to the bank. The Pops Concert is a new venture.

Within a half hour or so at this very nice affair, everyone felt honored, and there was no distinction between the "formals" and the "informals."
—*Janice Doherty in "Town and Country," a column on the society pages of the* Maine Sunday Telegram, *April 7, 1968*

of the latter, "Perspective," is now available in a 29-minute film, which can be shown to interested groups. . . .

In addition, the department has been most fortunate in gaining the interest and cooperation of the Department of Maine, American Legion, the American Legion Auxiliary, and the individual posts. Through the Legion's effort and support Pineland was able to obtain a 54-passenger bus for the children, and though the Legion Auxiliary's original "Wheelchair Fund" was only aimed at contributing ten wheelchairs for the benefit of otherwise bed-fast patients, this drive snowballed to such an extent that we should end up by being able to double this number. . . .

The department has also been fortunate in obtaining the cooperation of many businesses and entertainment firms, through which free merchandise has been donated or free entertainment provided. . . .

The department has conducted many tours of the Institution for various groups ranging from 1 to 75 members, including the Maine Congressional Delegation, and all other people interested in Pineland.

As a trial in the new Socialization Program, the girls of Doris Sidwell Hall have been granted permission to walk or bike ride on any of the roads of Pineland within reason. The girls have also been granted permission to visit the yards and porches of any building if the aides on duty in these buildings are agreeable. If the aides of any building wish to invite D.S.H. girls into a building to visit, they may do so if D.S.H. is notified in each instance.

D.S.H. is extending an invitation to any boy friendly with a D.S.H. girl (only on a one-to-one basis) to visit with his building superior's permission in the living room or recreation room [at very specific and limited hours]. The boys may bring records, games, etc. with them but are not to leave them in D.S.H. on completion of the visit. On Sundays, an invitation may possibly be made for a few of the boys to have supper with the girls. . . .

—Pineland Observer, *November 1970*

Throughout the 1950s and 1960s, the *Observer* would be an informative and entertaining vehicle for passing news around the institution and beyond. Begun as a monthly in 1953, the publication had, in its first editions, hand-drawn covers and articles ranging from official Bowman pronouncements to homey notes about recipes and holidays. When workers left for employment beyond the grounds—and sometimes even in other buildings on the grounds—the fond good-byes of those left behind were included in the *Observer*. When residents encountered skunks and employees encountered accidents and illnesses, the *Observer* was quick to make note. When Hoffman and other researchers at the school completed studies, the *Observer* reported the results.

The paper would grow and change with Pineland. Photographs would replace drawings on the covers, and type styles would grow increasingly sophisticated. In the 1970s, the monthly would become a bimonthly, then a quarterly. By the 1990s, it would shrink to a few typeset pages with a professional look and a distinct public relations touch. But for now the *Observer* was thick and rich and homespun.

In 1963, Moore summarized his department's early efforts, saying, "[I]t is felt by this department that, because of its many and varied activities, much of Maine's population—formerly having little knowledge of Pineland Hospital and its activities—is now at least reasonably well-acquainted with our hospital and programs."

That success was no cause to slow down, however, and the earnest activity of the department continued. In 1965 the state's television viewers were treated to a view of Thanksgiving dinner in one of the hospital's cottages as well as a clip of Pineland's Christmas pageant.

The public relations department was always quick to report Pineland's good news, such as the creation of Tall Pines, a day camp begun with financial help from the Volunteers of Pineland Fund, Inc., based on proceeds from "Pineland Pops" concerts played by the Portland Symphony Orchestra.

But digging out news of Pineland problems was a job more often left to others.

The Severely Retarded

By the late 1960s, Pineland had made considerable progress in its programs for the educable retarded. It had done much less for the profoundly retarded. In truth, hospitals such as Pineland could not do much for the most severe cases, Bowman argued at a 1969 legislative hearing on a bill that would require discharge of patients "medically judged to have maximally benefitted from the institution's care." Bowman said the idea was "common sense," and that for the severely retarded "protective lifelong care can be much more meaningfully given in a nursing home or boarding home where there is an easy chair, where they have potted plants in windows, which the large dehumanizing institution does not offer." Members of Pineland Parents and Friends disagreed with Bowman at the hearing, and the proposal died. But its consideration helped begin a debate that would echo through the halls of Pineland for three decades to come.

At this point, the news media had already begun a new round of Pineland investigations and exposés, some of them focusing on the care of the profoundly retarded at Pineland's Kupelian Hall.

"If you have a good staff-patient ratio you can teach even the lowest cases some toilet-training and feeding," Mrs. [Dorothy] Doyle [a Pineland nurse] said.

But the diminished staff at Pineland has so much to do that "toilet-training and teaching them to feed themselves is out of the question." . . .

In Kupelian Hall, she said, a lot of the patients must be tied in bed.

"You tell me how you're going to untie 80 or 90 patients when a fire breaks out," she said.

This problem could be largely eliminated, she said, if buildings such as Kupelian were equipped with crib-type instead of conventional beds. But Pineland has been unable to convince the powers that be in Augusta of this need.

—Brunswick Times Record, *July 20, 1967*

> As of July 1, 1970, all Psychiatric Aides I and II and Psychiatric Aide Supervisors I will no longer be required to wear a uniform. The following guidelines shall be followed:
> 1. Suitable clothing should be selected, keeping in mind the kind of patient and kind of activity going on for the day.
> 2. Washable clothing should be worn if at all possible. In the event clothing is worn which requires dry cleaning, a washable smock should be worn over all.
> 3. Good grooming will be expected at all times.
> —Pineland Observer, *February 1970*

Kenneth H. Morrison wrote one for *The Bath-Brunswick Times-Record* of Thursday, July 20, 1967. The story ran with a discomforting front-page photograph showing severely retarded patients outside the building, at least one in restraints, and all confined by a chain-link fence. The story said in part:

The building is dignified by having a name, Kupelian Hall. But it's really just a urine-fouled repository for the severely retarded—a throwback to the snakepits of old, different only in its modern trappings. . . .

All state institutions have serious problems, usually attributable to a shortage of funds.

Pineland, overcrowded and understaffed, has more than just serious problems on its hands. It has a major breakdown in services that has already reached scandalous proportions.

It should be stated at the outset that this breakdown has occurred in spite of the long hours and dedication of the hospital's hard-core administration and staff.

The cause-effect relationship of the problems at Pineland is almost too simple—deteriorating conditions due to a shortage of personnel, due to low salaries and near-impossible working conditions.

The shortage of personnel is a general problem that has placed a strain on just about all of its programs at Pineland, but it is at its most critical point and most observable in the caring for the "custodial" patients. The hospital has managed somehow to keep its programs for the "educable" and "trainable" retarded and for the emotionally disturbed from disintegrating. In fact, to tour Doris Sidwell Hall (a halfway house where girls are being prepared to return to the outside world) and to meet its residents is heartening and heartwarming.

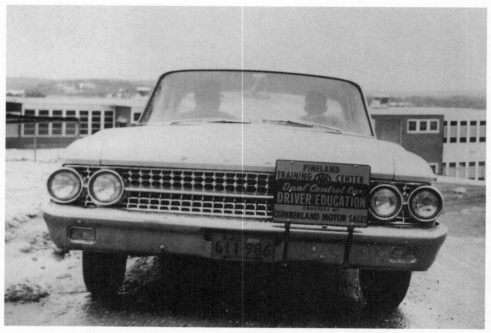

Pineland's driver training vehicle (courtesy of the New Gloucester Historical Society)

Kupelian Hall, however, is another story. And the human stench that emanates from it indicates the magnitude of the breakdown.

Hannah Kamber wrote a series of articles for the *Maine Times* in the winter and spring of 1969. She described the terrible conditions of Kupelian, with naked patients wandering aimlessly through the filth and smell of their own excrement, then compared it to the newly renovated Bliss Hall:

> *It would be impossible to describe the gross disparity between Kupelian Hall and Bliss Vocational Rehabilitation Center. One must see both. Twin buildings, the best and worst of Pineland's living halls for the retarded, they stand side by side at the rear of the grounds.*
>
> *The kindest thing I heard Kupelian called was "a virtual pigpen." Yet in Bliss, with its immaculate bedrooms and beautifully equipped classrooms, I saw a copy of* House Beautiful *displayed on an end table.*
>
> *The difference cannot be explained only in terms of higher and lower patient IQ, or by bricks and mortar renovation, or even by total funds and skill invested. In Bliss the patients are cared for as human beings, with the needs and potential for growth that are part of the human condition. In*

> [L]ast January in the adult females ward up to 30 out of 50 had to be restrained (tied, isolated, etc.) to prevent them from brutalizing their own and others' bodies.
>
> Now, after a program begun last June, which divided this female ward from a 50 patient unit into two 25 patient units, only four or five have to be periodically restrained.
>
> In June, 28 out of the 47 women trained could not feed themselves. Now there are only five non-feeders.
>
> In June, 47 out of 47 were not toilet-trained. Now all but 10 are completely trained.
>
> And, until the Work Activities Program was introduced, these women had never had an organized activity in all their lives.
>
> —Maine Times, *October 31, 1969*

Kupelian, excepting one unit, they are not; and its locked wards become another example of what has been called "the land of the living dead."

Editors and reporters sometimes tried to help as well as criticize. When Dr. Albert Anderson, Jr., director of program development, started a work activities program in which residents of Kupelian Hall could earn money (and, during training, marshmallows) by fitting wooden handles into mallet heads, Kamber and the *Maine Times* presented a positive report intended to help build voter support for a 1969 referendum question that would provide $350,000 for the Kupelian renovation—a question that eventually passed.

"Saints For Hire: 4¢ Per Hour," said the headline over a *Telegram* column by Bill Caldwell in September 1967. Chiding state legislators for failing to increase staff pay, he told of a ward orderly, Leo Small, who "has 44 very large children" to care for.

He feeds them; puts them on toilets; changes their clothes; helps wash them; helps comfort them; he gets them up, and he puts them to bed. All of them are grown men—far bigger than he is. "My kids," he calls them. Most of them cannot call him anything. They cannot talk. But Small can tell when they hurt, when they are sick, when they need the warmth of a hand clasp, when weird fear panics their galloping hearts. . . .

I look at Small's overtime card. This month he put in 80 hours of overtime, at straight time pay. No bonus at all except that the "kids," the helpless grown-up, loving kids, were not left alone. "But that is more than 2 weeks of overtime work in a four week month," I say.

There's only one bath tub and one makeshift shower in the women's wing. For 86 patients. But the patients don't care. They're not aware that they're jammed into a day room suitable for 25, or that they sleep in Flander's Field rows of cots in an adjoining community dormitory.

They don't care that many of their fellow inmates have to be fastened to their cots each night partly for their own protection and partly because there's only one psychiatric aide to watch over all of them.

Who does care? Their parents?

Statistics compiled on 355 random patients indicate that more than half had no visitors at all in 1966. Only 13 percent had one visit last year, nearly ten percent had two visits, and 4.6 percent had three. Only 14 of the group had ten or more visits.

Who does care? The volunteers?

Last year, of some 200 citizens who dedicate hours from their busy schedules to retarded patients at Pineland, only six—high school pupils from Gray and New Gloucester and a Bates College student—worked in Hayden Infirmary.

Not a single volunteer could face the bedlam, stench and the soul-searing sights in Kupelian Hall. But then, some of the regular workers at Pineland have never been there either.

Who cares? The attendants, the psychiatric aides who start at a $67 salary for a 44 hour week and will earn $90 after they've been there 15 years, only no one's ever stayed that long?

Yes, they care. Some work 12-16 hours a day at straight-time pay because they care. They never have help enough and the situation worsens every year. . . .

—*Hazel Loveitt in* Maine Sunday Telegram, *September 10, 1967*

Small smiles. "You can add," he says. "The kids can't."

Pineland did not deny the problems revealed by such stories. The *Observer*, in fact, reprinted some in their entirety. Eager to use any opportunity for Pineland's benefit, Bowman stated for the Kamber series that Maine had done more for the retarded than some other states, and was "ahead of the national average in terms of community facilities." But, he added:

> *The continued existence of "snakepits" is a sad reflection on our confused value system that has come under fire in recent years.*

Why is it possible in Sweden and Denmark to replace "snakepits" with well-designed, attractively decorated functional structures where trained, kind, and well-paid personnel radiate friendliness and confidence—a far cry from our harassed, overworked and underpaid psychiatric aides at Kupelian Hall?

Why is it that we engage in public prayer meetings but avoid human misery under our very eyes?

The World According to Bowman

Once again, Bowman was being very, very sure that his thoughts were plainly heard. As Pappanikou said years later, "Peter wasn't ever afraid of fighting the establishment."

A year before, the superintendent had made headlines by speaking of death as a right and questioning the use, said the *Maine Sunday Telegram*, "of extraordinary medical efforts for terminal heart and cancer patients, the profoundly retarded, persons suffering decerebration as the result of excessive brain damage caused by accidents, and even Siamese twins whose heads are fused, with no hope for a meaningful life."

Total number of residents benefitting from the Recreation Program: 1,063

Maximum rate of parental support for patients: $14 per week

Number of panes of glass replaced daily: as many as 32

Number of boys employed working with the groundsman mowing lawns and shoveling: 15

Number of meals served each day: between 4,700 and 4,800

Pounds of laundry processed each day: 5,000

Gallons of water used daily: 200,000

Valley Farm piggery population: 166 pigs and hogs

Acres planted at the Hill Farm: 40

Hay cut by Hill and Valley crews: 400 tons

Number of birds that could be handled by the poultry laying house: 4,000

Distance of the Collier Brook water source: 2.5 miles

Kilowatt hours of electricity generated daily: 4,000

Barrels of fuel oil consumed every day: 100

Gallons of hot water used hourly by the laundry: 4,000

Pounds of steam generated daily: more than 400,000

—Pownal Observer, *May 1966*

A month after that, Bowman defended the practice of forced sterilization for retarded women who kept bearing illegitimate children. Maine was then one of five states allowing such procedures, though it was used no more than five times a year, Bowman said.

In May 1970, Bowman leveled another angry blast at his employer, the state, telling the Lewiston-Auburn Rotary Club that the system supporting hospitals such as Pineland was "hopelessly inadequate, antiquated and unresponsive. . . . State government continues to plow with oxen when everyone else uses a tractor."

Pineland had won accreditation after a decade of hard work, but the Augusta State Hospital had lost its accreditation and the Bangor State Hospital had never received it. "This reflects gross professional negligence and lack of candor in the first degree," he told the Rotarians. "It also reflects lack of concern by you, because you—through your elected representative—have the ultimate responsibility for conditions that should no longer be tolerated."

Such charges made many headlines, fewer friends. The powers in Augusta were beginning to stir.

The State Strikes Back

The state bureaucracy had reconfigured itself since the time of Kupelian, and the department now responsible for Pineland was the Department of Mental Health and Corrections. Led since 1969 by Commissioner William F. Kearns, Jr., the department had limited control over Bowman, whose position was tenured through the civil service system.

That changed abruptly with legislative passage of a law giving the commissioner the power to appoint superintendents and administrators of the department's institutions. Kearns said that when the law took effect in September 1971, he would

---

"DO YOU KNOW WHY THE WHISTLE BLOWS AT 11:25 A.M.?"

Among other queries the Library received recently, was the question posed above.

A phone call to the Power House elicited the answer that it was to let Berman School know it was time to end classes for lunch time.

A call to the school then established that classes didn't end until noon. When they were asked if they knew why the whistle blew at 11:25, if it wasn't for their benefit, they readily replied that it was to let Engineering know it was time to pack up their tools and to go to lunch!

—Pineland Observer, *October 1970*

> Six years have passed at Pineland
> Since Doctor Bowman came
> The changes and new buildings
> Things are not the same
> The place was always pitiful
> The children's look forlorn.
> Now when I go to see them
> That look is past and gone.
> Children act more friendly now
> I know they see the change
> They speak and smile and wave good-bye
> Since Doctor Bowman came.
>
> —Pineland Observer, *June 1959, from a ten-verse*
> *poem "Contributed by a Friend"*

not reappoint Bowman. "Outspoken Pineland Super Out of Job" reported the leading headline in the *Portland Press Herald* on July 21 of that year.

Bowman reacted loudly and often. He had been "sideswiped," he said. He had many options but no intention to leave. He would fight the decision in court—and he did, for several years.

Various newspapers recounted Bowman's more controversial statements and recalled his frequent open disputes with Kearns. A *Press Herald* columnist mentioned that Kearns had taken some of the superintendent's public complaints personally, and that Bowman and a senior member of the department had disagreed so intensely about a question on patient safety that the other man challenged Bowman to go outside and fight.

Many defenders leapt to Bowman's side, including 225 state workers who roared their support in a standing ovation, according to press accounts. Defenders also included former governor Frederick G. Payne, many parents and friends of Pineland residents, and several legislators, including Thomas L. Maynard of Weld, who said in a letter to the *Press Herald* that Maine ought to promote and not fire the man who had dragged Pineland "out of the darkness of the nineteenth century."

But such sentiment would not prevail, and the courts would reject every attempt to reverse the state's position. Bowman's Pineland career was done.

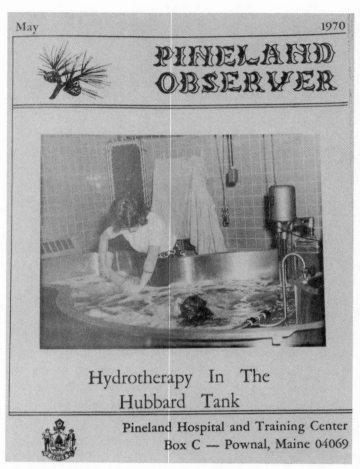

May   1970

PINELAND OBSERVER

Hydrotherapy In The
Hubbard Tank

Pineland Hospital and Training Center
Box C — Pownal, Maine 04069

Pineland Observer, *May 1970 (courtesy of the New Gloucester Historical Society)*

Division and Consent: The 1970s 5

*Progress everywhere today does seem to come so very
heavily disguised as Chaos.*
                                    —Joyce Grenfell

"We have reached a crossroad in our evolution that requires reflection, reorientation, and redefinition of purposes and goals," said Superintendent Peter W. Bowman in 1963.

The doctor understated the case. His simple "crossroad" was actually a major, fluctuating interchange that occupied a space in time extending through decades. People, trends, treatments, laws, philosophies, and passions sped into the Pineland interchange from myriad directions, merged and mixed for a bit, sometimes colliding like so many bumper cars, then shot off along their separate ways, perhaps to disappear forever, perhaps to reemerge and converge again in different times and different ways.

The decade of the 1970s was at the center of the interchange, a period when major new forces from outside the state merged and mixed with those inside. Across America, retardation was now openly acknowledged as a condition found at every level of society. Disabilities in general were a cause attracting the nation's attention and resources.

Private organizers across the land were continuing to build the Special Olympics movement begun with the first games in Chicago on July 20, 1968. Those, said Special Olympics, Inc., on its Web page in the year 2000, were "the beginning of a worldwide movement to demonstrate that people with mental retardation are capable of remarkable achievements in sports, education, employment, and beyond."

Congress continued its involvement in 1970 by amending the Mental Retardation Facilities and Community Mental Health Centers Construction Act of

It seems strange, for the third month in a row, to put together our Pineland Observer without making any comment on the current managerial crisis. But the in-fighting is so intense, many of us are pulled so strongly one way or another, that with your Editor's feelings so wholeheartedly on one side of the issue, her judgment is undoubtedly biased.

Thus, since we cannot be neutral and report completely objectively on what's happening, so rather than add fuel to the already blazing conflagration, we shall continue to omit newspaper references to the situation. Again, for those who wish to see the newspaper stories not reprinted in this Observer, the Scrapbook in the Administration Building is open for perusal.

But the important thing for all of us to remember is that Pineland now is under heavy scrutiny because of all the publicity, and we must not let ourselves be sidetracked from our primary responsibility—

"To afford the very best care and treatment we can to Pineland's residents"—by factional party loyalty.

No matter how the conflict resolves itself, it cannot be allowed to diminish the services we are offering to handicapped individuals entrusted to our care.

"Hold the good thought!"

—*Rose Ricker, editor,* Pineland Observer, *November 1973,*
after the firing of Dr. Peter W. Bowman, superintendent

1963, and in 1975 by passing the Education for All Handicapped Children Act. Funds produced by such legislation grew rapidly through time; in 1985, $1.1 billion would go to a variety of programs that would help mainstream children previously served in institutions such as Pineland and in the segregated special education classes of public schools.

Terminology was changing again, too. In 1973, the American Association on Mental Deficiency rewrote its definition of "mental retardation." Now the category included people whose IQs were two deviations from the norm, not just the one previously used as the measure. Children once called "mildly retarded" or "educable retarded" were now "children with learning disabilities." Academic though they might sound, these new approaches had a profound impact on individual lives, said James W. Trent, Jr., in *Inventing the Feeble Mind*: "As the change in definition accompanied changes in consciousness and funding, many people who had been officially

When High School Basketball Tournaments were being publicized and played by teams throughout the state, there was another special, but less visible, basketball tournament in the making—the New England Basketball Tournament for the Mentally Retarded in Hartford—one of the largest tournaments ever involving a Maine team.

What had made this tournament so significant was that it involved a special population of people who are usually deprived of such privileges and luxuries; a population seldom given credit when due, either because of their seemingly unimportant accomplishments or because their feats may seem secondary to others. . . .

The Pineland Chargers and their cheerleaders displayed such an overwhelming desire to attend such a tournament that it left no alternative but to make an effort and get the money to send them and their faithful supporters to Connecticut. . . .

During the week of March 15-19, nine boys and three girls began their trip to Hartford, where they resided for the week at the Holiday Inn. Accommodations were very appropriate and a definite change from the usual institutional environment. The tournament was held at nearby Trinity College.

Several states throughout New England sent a total of 22 teams and their cheerleaders... Pineland was placed in Division 4 and won a 1st place trophy.

Pineland Chargers and their cheerleaders, Maine's sole representatives, not only brought home victory, but more importantly returned with the respect of others because of their sportsmanship, friendship, and cooperation with other team members. . . .

> —*Raymond Caouette, member of Pineland's recreation department*, Maine Sunday Telegram, *April 25, 1976*

considered mentally retarded were by the end of the decade freed from the label and from the accompanying structures of state control."

From across the Atlantic came a new term for the retardation cause. Imported from Scandinavia, "normalization," in the words of Trent, was "elevated to a principle" by Wolf Wolfensberger, a Nebraska psychologist who led "an apostolic campaign to denounce state schools and to establish the community as the sole locus of services for retarded citizens."

The word "normalization" fit Pineland's evolving ideas just right and soon echoed about the changing brick halls. "The renovation of our unit has meant another step forward in normalization for the profoundly retarded children," said a 1972 report on a renovation of Kupelian Hall in the *Observer*. "The day hall is spacious," the article continued, giving distinct local meaning to the term:

> *We have girls who were previously sitting by themselves with no desire to join in the fun of play, dancing, or even walking without an aide to tell them, who are now blooming into individuals who are letting us really know they are there. One girl who spent years in a state of depression, not caring to be included in the fun of any of the activities is now dancing and laughing and getting all she can out of everything and everyone around her.*

Within the state, the movements toward deinstitutionalization and wider involvement in Pineland's affairs continued. Gone with Bowman were the days when one man could firmly lead Maine's responses to and discussions about retardation from his office on the isolated campus of Pineland. Now many others were grabbing for the reins the state had yanked from Bowman's grasp. Parent groups,

---

It takes $5,000 a year to keep someone at Pineland. If the state gave this money to parents of retarded children to buy residential care, I think it would improve our system. I'm quite sure they wouldn't purchase the services of our state residential centers.

Our society is based on elite control of the handicapped rather than on provision for them.

It becomes a relationship of he is sick and I am well and therefore I know best so I'm going to tell him. In fact he may have much better ways to make himself well.

—*Dr. Albert Anderson, Jr., 1971*

Pineland Parents and Friends, an association made up largely of parents of retarded children in the hospital and training center here, is circulating petitions seeking to prevent the transfer of patients to nursing and boarding homes.

Marcel Michaud of Lewiston, president of the association, said . . . he expects to get at least 2,000 signers and intends to put the petitions before the special legislative session next month.

—Portland Press Herald, *December 17, 1971*

patient advocates, labor unions, legislators, Augusta administrators, and staff members all spoke up, often in loud voices dutifully recorded by a press that increasingly used phrases such as "the cloud of controversy" and "Pineland's woes" to describe affairs at the school.

As in the past, some news reports were lengthy, considered exposés, in the manner of the *Maine Times* articles of 1969. Others intended to praise. "Pineland Center Has Come A Long Way In 65 Years" said the *Lewiston Evening Journal*, offering a full-page history centered on an open house at the school in October 1973. That June, the same paper had offered another full-page article, this one focused on Pineland's famed Independence Day celebrations. Still other news reports responded to daily events on the campus, such as athletic contests, staff changes, and volunteer teas.

A Telling Report

The Church World: Maine's Official Catholic Weekly presented one of the decade's more thoughtful journalistic appraisals of the institution. Written and photographed in 1972 by John Kerry, diocesan research director of social legislation, "The plight of Maine's mentally retarded" appeared first in series and then as a newsprint booklet of sixteen 11- by 17-inch pages. Said the cover text:

> *Pineland Hospital and Training Center is universally recognized as one of the nation's outstanding institutions for the treatment and training of the mentally retarded. It offers progressive programs in speech and physical therapy, occupational and vocational training, recreation and education. Yet does it, as a residential institution, provide an appropriate environment for maximum rehabilitation? For instance, does the infirmary . . . offer a vestige of hope to retarded individuals who deserve the chance to develop and contribute their abilities to society, or are they doomed to forgotten lives in an institution as societal rejects?*

In the aftermath of Vietnam, people couldn't protest against that so they had to find other things to protest. Pineland became a target for that as did many other facilities. . . . Institutions became politically incorrect. . . . Eventually there was a general perception that Pineland was an unacceptable facility.

—Dr. H. Jay Monroe, acting superintendent in the 1970s, looking back in the year 2000

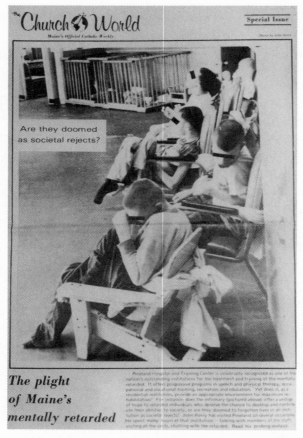

The Church World, *1972 (courtesy of the New Gloucester Historical Society, with permission of* The Church World)

Kerry had spent considerable time on the campus before writing about what he saw, he would recall in January 2001. "I stayed overnight sometimes, and moved around to all the buildings. Nobody had ever done that before, and I learned a lot because in some of the buildings, the patients stayed very active at night." He was motivated, he said, by religious commitment. His purpose was not writing an exposé but showing the people of Pineland as human beings, "because even the retarded are children of God."

His interest was personally rewarding, he added. "This was a very profound experience for me. A moving experience."

Kerry concluded his series with a call for more community services along with more specialized programs at Pineland for retarded individuals with extraordinary disabilities. Working toward those proposals with his own writing, he provided a useful and independent if personal assessment of Maine's retarded population and programs. There were said to be 30,000 retarded persons in the state, he reported. Fewer than 800 were in institutions such as Pineland, and only 400 were profoundly retarded. In fact, "27,000 are educable and could live productive and independent lives in the community if the proper resources were available."

Social attitudes toward retardation were improving, Kerry said, but at a painfully slow pace:

> Slowly, very slowly, the stigma of retardation is being removed from its niche in our social standards. People are less apt to ridicule, criticize and ostracize the mentally retarded as was the case in years past. Yet, we have just begun; and we have a long way to go before our uninformed and emotional prejudices are removed and replaced by humanistic values—that will respect each individual person in Maine regardless of his IQ, whether it be 200 or 20.

The state's response to retardation was also changing, Kerry noted. A new Bureau of Mental Retardation had been created within the Department of Mental Health and Corrections. Its director was Dr. Albert Anderson, Jr., who had previously developed new programs for the profoundly retarded at Pineland. Anderson believed that institutions such as Pineland were outmoded, and that the bureau should extend its efforts beyond Pineland. So the bureau was hiring regional coordinators to build services for the retarded throughout the state. It was also supporting the Elizabeth Levinson Developmental Center in Bangor, a new state-of-the-art facility funded by the legislature in 1971 "to let the mentally retarded obtain an existence as close to the normal as possible [by] making available to them patterns and conditions of everyday life which are as close as possible to the norms of society." Kerry's photos of Levinson showed identifiable youngsters in typical kids' clothing and contrasted sharply with his photos of Pineland, many of them featuring profoundly retarded adults in the infirmary, some in diapers, some in one-size-for-all institutional suits of nylon, most with their eyes blocked by the printer with black bands of ink to shield their identity.

The Levinson Center impressed Kerry, who called it "in all probability, the closest approximation to the best our country can offer to our mentally retarded citizens at the present time." Perhaps, he continued, the center would allay the fears of parents concerned about the possibility of moving state services from Pineland into such community-based facilities.

Kerry wrote of the anguish of parents faced with placing their children in Pineland, of the anger of some at the treatment of their children there, and of the gratitude of others, who considered the place "a God-send and a blessing."

Mrs. Walker [Theresa, a former Pineland patient] continued to be extremely frightened and agitated during the questions. It came out later that she had been upset and sleepless since receiving the letter [asking for an interview]. She had set a definite date so that she wouldn't have to wait any longer. Both Hubby and Johnny [a friend] had attempted to calm her about this visit. She was worried that she would not "pass the test" and be taken back to [Pineland]. She stated that she had been there for some twenty years and did not ever want to go back. I assured her that there was no test and there was no possibility of her going back. It was not until I repeated this some ten times that she seemed at ease.

>   —*An interview reported in John L. Hoffman's study*
>   *of former Pineland residents. Names were*
>   *changed for the report.*

Theresa was married to Richard Walker, also a former Pineland resident. She had entered the institution in 1940 at age nineteen, after a troubled period in her life, and stayed until 1958. "These two appear to have made an excellent adjustment," the report concluded.

Richard Walker was born in 1907. Admitted in 1919 at age 12. . . . The background on this case is one of the most obscure. Richard came [to Pineland] from an orphanage, and his placement here was apparently without justification. Illegitimacy and assiduous concealment are not impossible, with Richard as victim. On discharge, after 35 years of institutional life, he wrote, "It seems as though I am coming out of a dream and left it way behind."

>   —*An interview reported in John L. Hoffman's study*
>   *of former Pineland residents, published in 1969.*
>   *Names were changed for the report. Richard later*
>   *married Theresa (Redding) Walker, another*
>   *former resident.*

He wrote of the worst at the Pineland of 1972—the infirmary, "the dumping place for the mentally retarded," the "end of the line," according to one staff member, with its "dehumanizing sterility," its "stomach turning odors," its most difficult patients, some deformed, some restrained in chairs or tied to walls or beds. He also wrote of what seemed to him the best at Pineland, the Hospital Improvement Program, funded by the federal Department of Health and Welfare and designed to train children for a return to the community. That program enjoyed a patient-staff ratio of 8:1 (the same as at the Levinson Center), he observed, instead of the 20:1 or higher ratios found elsewhere at the school. And he identified other solid efforts that "are invaluable to a great many retarded individuals," such as "vocational rehabilitation, speech, physical, and hearing therapy, educational, medical, and dental programs, as well as a variety of recreational and personal services."

Kerry offered sympathy to parents for the confusion they must be feeling. Maine physicians had long offered Pineland as the only solution for retarded children. "Yet, after years of struggling to get their mentally retarded children into Pineland, parents are now being told that Pineland is not the ideal place for them and that they should be seeking other solutions. . . . The advice, oddly enough, is not coming from enlightened social reformers or institutional critics, but from the administrators and staff at Pineland Hospital and Training Center." Dr. H. Jay Monroe, one of two interim superintendents to serve after the firing of Dr. Bowman, was one of the administrators. He told Kerry:

> *The mentally retarded individuals are persons and they deserve the rights and privileges of every other citizen. They have physical, emotional and psycho-social needs that must and can be met if they are given the opportunity. Many people feel that the mentally retarded cannot be helped. They are wrong. They can be helped if given the chance. We feel that the needs of most mentally retarded persons can best be met in the community, not in an institution such as Pineland. We can provide quality services for some of the mentally retarded, not all. Our goal is not to keep people here forever; it's to help prepare them for their return to the community.*

Another strong and prophetic statement came to Kerry from Dr. Saul Niedorf, director of psychiatric services:

> *The Legislature has passed laws and now they are currently violating the law. They have not provided us with the money or personnel resources*

A great many employees at Pineland Center have been mired in pessimism and paranoia for the past few years. Many of us have been sickened and disheartened by the loss of standards or the lack of adhering to present policies.

—Nancy L. Wilcox, beginning a five-page letter stating specific complaints to John Rosser, Ed.D., commissioner of Mental Health and Corrections, April 9, 1975.

Community volunteers have entertained at the Walter J. Soucy Gymnasium and in many buildings throughout the year. The variety and caliber of visiting performers are commendable, ranging from solo appearances by an Easter Bunny to a two-hour presentation by the Symphony String Quartet. Organizations generously give parties throughout the year, and every holiday has been appropriately celebrated with their support.
—*Volunteer Services annual report, June 30, 1972*

they have promised. I'm a physician and I believe in the medical model; I think by it and I live by it. I will welcome the day when someone sues us for the type of care and treatment our patients are getting here at Pineland.

The Caring Side of Pineland

In January 2001, Kevin Concannon, Maine's commissioner of Human Services, recalled the Kerry series as "the most determinate" journalistic report of the period, a report that helped shape Pineland's history. Concannon himself was deeply involved in that history, as an acting superintendent in the late 1970s and again in the late 1980s, and in various other prominent government roles. "What John Kerry had to say was compelling and very powerful," he said. *The Church World* had a circulation of about 20,000 at the time, and its recipients included every legislator in Augusta. "So that series helped change things."

For all its value, Kerry's report, like many others of the decade, focused on problems and the need for change. It gave less attention to the caring side of Pineland, the side steadily and quietly personified by its many committed staff members and volunteers.

Joseph M. Ferri saw that side. He had gone to work at Pineland as a teacher in 1964. One of many long-term Pineland workers, he would stay for three decades in various capacities, including a short stint as superintendent in the 1980s.

"There were problems of course," he said, looking back in the year 2000. One was based in the fact of trainable residents earning union wages at places such as Hillcrest Poultry Company.

That meant they were literally making more money than the staff. That was a problem. And as the more capable people moved out, there were fewer people to help care for the profoundly retarded, to clean up the messes on the floor, things like that.

But you know, there were a lot of good dedicated people on the staff. They used to get hurt because everything said about the place was negative, especially in the newspapers. You knew how much they cared because they were always taking patients home for holidays and cooking things for them and bringing those in. They knew what the children liked and they provided it out of their own pockets. This sort of thing happened all the time.

Sometimes people say that was a bad place to work, and I say "then ask me why I stayed there thirty years." It was a good place to work. Every day you did not know what you would be doing. It always kept me motivated and interested. Some of those people took a long time to learn things, but when they did, the staff felt very good. There were definitely some real positives.

Conrad P. Lausier found positives, too. He and his wife both worked at Pineland, he as an ambulance driver and she as an aide, then as an office clerk. Five of the Lausiers' nine children also found jobs at Pineland at various times. "From my point of view it was a godsend for me," he said, remembering back from the year 2000. It helped with the bills—especially when the family had seven children in college at once. Ten years of work there led Lausier and his wife to better-paying jobs with the Department of Human Services in Portland. And while Lausier was

---

Several aides at Kupelian Hall III got together and decided that it might be different to take some of their most severely handicapped residents on a shopping trip in the community.

Five young men were selected (partially because they did have money in their own accounts, but principally because—as far as anyone knew—none of them had ever been in a store in their lives before).

K-Mart in Falmouth was the store selected, and Bob Arsenault reports that the employees there could not have been more helpful or understanding. . . .

After their buying spree the boys were all treated to a McDonald's supper. Everyone seemed to have a grand time, and the boys were, on the whole, very well behaved. Bob says they plan to have other shopping trips in the future, and also that he hopes to be able to take a group to the wrestling matches at the Expo.

—Pineland Observer, *February 1973*

at Pineland, he had lots of freedom, a chance to move around on the grounds and well beyond, plus an opportunity "to get to know the kids."

There were adventures, too. Once Lausier was driving a patient south from Bangor to Pineland in an ambulance when he came across an accident involving a truck carrying horses. "God, what a hell of a mess," he said. The Pineland patient got in the front seat with Lausier, who put the truck driver into the rear of the ambulance and headed back to Bangor. On another occasion, Lausier had to take a patient to a Boston hospital. He had been to Massachusetts only once before and had no idea where the hospital was. So he found a cab parked at the side of the road and paid the driver to lead him to his destination.

Lausier was a more frequent visitor to Maine hospitals, and he stored strait-jackets at the Maine Medical Center in case he needed them for transporting difficult patients. Occasionally he could give the hospital staff helpful information about his patients. "You're wasting your time," he told a nurse who was digging out pajamas for a young boy whom Lausier had brought in. "Sure enough, the next day they called and said 'come on over and get him,' and egad, when I got there he'd torn all the sheets up and he had no clothes on him at all."

Pineland helped some of Lausier's patients. "One kid was so crippled she couldn't even walk. She had a spine thing. But I took her in for a bunch of operations and one day I saw her walking from her building to the canteen. Egad it was wonderful. I never thought I'd see it." Still, things weren't perfect, said Lausier.

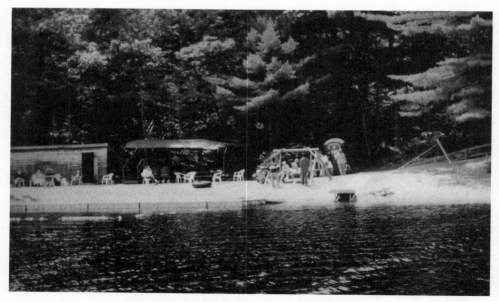

Tall Pines Day Camp (courtesy of the New Gloucester Historical Society)

Ernest [a former Pineland patient], much against the better sense and advice of his friends, has conceived an elaborate and irrational scheme whereby he can show by signs of manufactured stability and good behavior that his stay at the reformatory and Pineland should be stricken from the public records. . . .

Ernest is bitter about his stay at Pineland, not only because he didn't belong here but also because of the sneaky way he was transferred from the reformatory to the State School and spent seven years beyond his original sentence. Fixing a steady gaze on me he said, "I figure the state owes me those seven years."

—An interview reported in John L. Hoffman's study
of former Pineland residents, published in 1969.
Names were changed for the report. Ernest had
been transferred from the Men's Reformatory to
the Pownal State School in 1950 and remained
until 1955. The victim of a horrendous childhood
family situation, he led a troubled adult life after
his release.

Bowman "was no damn fool, I tell you," but he "didn't pay too much attention to the so-called low grades. It was mostly custodial for them, and egads, it was a hell of a mess."

Nancy L. Wilcox shared Lausier's view that Pineland was imperfect. She started at Pineland as a hospital aide in 1969 and eventually became a secretary in the Berman School. Overall "I really liked it," she said later. She also liked Bowman, although she almost got in trouble the first time they met. She did not know who he was or why he was talking to a patient, but she knew that the patient was in the wrong place, "so I marched up and said, 'you ought to be in school.'" Bowman did not object, but others felt differently when she voiced her concerns about problems at Pineland all the way up the chain of command to the governor. Once she complained about a state police officer's investigation of a car accident she had at the school. "I found out later that they put out an order to watch for my car. They said to 'get her for anything.'"

The volunteer effort at Pineland remained strong well into the decade. In the year ending on June 30, 1973, a total of 225 volunteers contributed 9,926 hours of time. Some of their accomplishments and other positive stories did reach the public. In 1972, for example, the Portland papers gave several columns of coverage to

Maine's Special Olympics. Other papers of the same year told of the developing Tall Pines Day Camp, new grants for Pineland researchers, new professional training programs, and the Sesame Street float that won Pineland residents a prize at Pownal's Old Home Days celebration. But for many readers, the positives were buried under other stories.

Boiling Passions

A period of intense ferment may have been inevitable as the forces of change pressed on in the early 1970s. Whether inevitable or not, the period was painful and prolonged.

When the Hichens committee made it known that they could be approached by institutional employees and utilized as a kind of legislative ombudsman that could defend the employee against the bureaucrats, the angry balloons began to burst.

Hichens was overwhelmed with phone calls, began seeing institutional workers in motel rooms, hearing rooms, at home, wherever and whenever he could. As their stories—often spiced by sparks from an old grudge—began piling up, Hichens began assembling the information he would use to bring permissive bureaucrats into line.

Like many preachers of virtue, Senator Hichens and several of his committee members have a special interest in sin; and, like many institutional workers, the employees have a particular fascination with gossip and scandal. The meetings between the two had predictable results. Rumors of sexual promiscuity at Pineland began making the rounds; the Stevens Home for Girls became a nest for lesbians; a juvenile experiment in coeducation became a teen-age orgy; drugs were being delivered weekly by the Mafia to the State Hospital and distributed through the network of tunnels under the buildings. And so on, as far as the imaginations of the story tellers and the eagerness of the listeners would take it.

But underneath the wild tales was a platform of honest complaints about the way the long-neglected institutions were being operated. There was some substance to the stories told to the Hichens committee, largely because they had never been able to be told before, and because no other group of any stature in Maine had ever taken a citizen interest in places like Pineland and Thomaston.

—*John N. Cole in* Maine Times, *April 13, 1973*

The ousted Dr. Bowman continued for several more years to make loud complaints and large headlines in his futile attempt to recover his job.

Alarmed that Pineland would release patients "who are beyond rehabilitation" into the community, Marcel Michaud, president of Pineland Parents and Friends, asked the group to consider buying Pineland from the state.

State senator Walter Hichens, a Republican from Eliot, attacked the school in 1972, charging it with "encouraging sexual freedom" through its Hospital Improvement Program, and setting off a debate about normalization and a new state probe of Pineland. The program did have a sex education component, said Dr. Monroe, then acting administrator at the school. He said that one patient at the school was pregnant and another had had an abortion, but "we certainly don't condone promiscuity."

The bureau chief in Augusta also responded to Hichens, denying that there was more promiscuity at Pineland than ever before. "But we're dealing with men and women, and sexual relations is a natural event . . . ," Anderson said. "Basically, we have a choice. If we want to lock everyone up, we would eliminate sexual behavior. This would be a denial of their rights to engage in sexual behavior."

Hichens had doubts about the whole concept of normalization. Pineland was "trying to push patients out into the community too fast," he said. The idea of sexual rights was especially troublesome, and he thought Pineland should prevent all sexual activity. How? "They used to get after them and punish them," he told Jim Brunelle of the *Maine Sunday Telegram*. "Oh, I don't mean real harsh punishment, but enough to discourage them."

Some of the young workers in the Hospital Improvement Program were stunned at such charges. They had joined the program with idealistic purposes, remembered one of them two decades after the fact. "We did talk to residents about protecting themselves sexually," said William David Barry, later a writer of Maine social history. "We thought we were supposed to be there to help people. Then suddenly there was a war about what we were doing. This was crazy."

But Hichens was neither satisfied nor finished with Pineland, and he was not about to declare peace. A month later he demanded, with the support of the Senate's Health and Institutional Services Committee, that Anderson be fired—a demand refused by William F. Kearns, Jr., commissioner of Mental Health and Corrections. Later that year, Hichens was at it again, this time sponsoring a bill supported by Pineland Parents and Friends. It was an unsuccessful attempt to create a board of trustees for Pineland and to give parents of patients a legal voice in its operation.

Union members were unhappy, too; in September 1972, members of the American Federation of State, County and Municipal Employees began picketing the school, protesting the policies and actions of Dr. Niedorf at the Children's Psychiatric Hospital.

Still another threat to Pineland appeared in the summer of 1972 when the Greater Portland Council of Governments proposed locating a landfill on state grounds adjacent to Pineland—an effort that would eventually be prevented by the town of New Gloucester. Then, late in 1972, new headlines told of a parent's complaint that Pineland aides had hit her seven-year-old son with paddles.

A New Superintendent

Into this angry atmosphere, in October 1972, stepped Dr. Bowman's replacement. He was Conrad R. Wurtz, Ph.D., previously a mental retardation official in Iowa. A psychologist, Wurtz was Pineland's first nonmedical superintendent. He was a quiet man, committed to the idea of deinstitutionalization and intent on letting "program instead of personality" control Pineland's agenda.

A building-by-building survey conducted early in his superintendency cataloged needs from toilet training to dish washing and revealed that there was much for both program and person to do. The statistics for the Cumberland Hall basement, for example, showed that all thirty-six residents were feeding themselves; thirty were completely toilet trained, but six were trained "day only"; and twenty-five were dressing themselves but eleven were not.

In Gray Hall, an employee spoke of major program needs:

In an effort to evade the typical, stodgy annual report, and to give a brief overview of the myriad changes effected in fiscal 1972-73, the following capsule narrative will provide the highlights of the year.

The dominating event which set the scene for what was to follow was, of course, the appointment in the fall of a new superintendent, Conrad R. Wurtz, Ph.D., the first non-medical superintendent in Pineland's almost 75-year-old history. Well-qualified, Dr. Wurtz came to Maine from Iowa, where he had been Director of the Bureau of Mental Retardation. With this drastic change in leadership came an equally drastic change in administrative attitudes and policies. From a strictly hierarchical, departmentalized institution, Pineland started evolving into an organization where participative management was encouraged and decision-making shared.

—*Pineland Hospital and Training Center annual report, June 30, 1973*

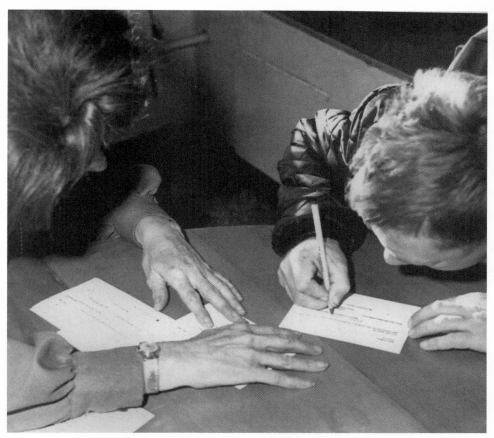

Writing lesson (courtesy of the Maine State Archives)

> *We are simply training the residents to sit quietly and do nothing in a more orderly and pleasant manner. Although urine and feces are no longer on the floor, although residents are all dressed, look relatively neat, eat orderly, do not holler and scream as much, THEY STILL BASICALLY SIT, HAVING NOTHING TO DO. We still act as wardens, guarding the inmates.*

And in Cumberland Hall there were physical problems:

> *Cumberland Hall II remains a unit which receives unwanted residents and undesirables in a broader sense from other buildings. Present major goals have changed little over the years; i.e., continuing the present program of improving activity of daily living skills. In addition, major goals involve placing the main emphasis upon lowering the census and upon*

improving the physical plant, e.g., removing a partition on Ward A, replac-
ing the tile on the bathroom floors, keeping one bathroom wall from cav-
ing in, replacing the leaky plumbing, etc. Dishes are rinsed in a slopsink in
the mop closet before being sent back to the kitchen. The newly installed
bathtub drains into the dishwasher in the basement.

Was Pineland a hornets' nest during his tenure? Wurtz was asked some years later. "Oh was it ever," he replied. His stay would be brief—about two and a half years. Some would see him as a fresh thinker, and some as ineffectual, but he was pleased by the significant developments of his stay. Among the first was a departure from the medical focus that had become so intense under Bowman. Arguing that emotionally disturbed children should be cared for in small live-in centers scattered around the state rather than at Pineland, Wurtz and administrators in Augusta phased out the Children's Psychiatric Hospital in 1973—despite protests from some legislators, parents, and union members.

The hospital had already lost the services of Dr. Niedorf, its controversial director. Niedorf's job was protected by civil service regulations. He could not be fired, but he could be banned from the hospital and reassigned to the Bureau of Mental Health in Augusta, and he was. After several highly publicized months of not running the hospital while continuing to receive one of the state's highest salaries for doing so, he resigned "in disgust and frustration."

The move from Pineland's medical focus was further marked in 1973 by passage of a legislative act dropping the hospital reference from its name; the institution now became known as Pineland Center.

Two years after that, the state would cut ties with Pineland's more distant farming past by transferring 1,159 acres of its land to the state's Bureau of Public Lands and leaving the center with 291 acres around its buildings.

In the meantime, Pineland was reorganizing the rest of its programs. A new "unitization" plan was designed to regroup patients according to their handicaps instead of their ages, and November 29, 1973, became "Moving Day," the date when

---

It was tough when the psychiatric hospital was closing. Another aide and I put a boy onto the elevator to send him downstairs. When the doors closed we both started crying and walking in opposite directions. We were losing our kids.

—*Wayne Haskell, psychiatric aide in Children's*
Psychiatric Hospital, remembering back in
the year 2000

My heart goes out to the wonderful supervisory personnel and daily contact aides who have worked their hearts and guts out not only for my child but for all the other darling children in Staples Hall whom I've grown to love during my monthly visits there. When Dr. Wurtz comes along with a stupid idea that only makes their jobs even more difficult, it makes me want to throw up.

—Letter to the Lewiston Sun *from a parent responding to unitization changes, December 14, 1973*

Despite the fact there is a wider range of ages now together in Staples Hall, there are a great number of benefits to be derived since they all need the same developmental training.

—Dr. Conrad Wurtz, Portland Evening Express, *December 20, 1973*

80 percent of Pineland's residents were shifted to new locations on campus. Some workers who assisted remembered that event as confused and close to traumatic, with occasional residents who had lost their identity tags being identified by names written on their foreheads with markers. The move done, new teams began working with residents in four different categories: primary development and training, for the most severely handicapped; child development, to help children get back into community schools; adult community living, to train adults for return to the larger community; and vocational training and special services. The changes, said Wurtz, would allow individual training for residents and advance "the ultimate goal," to "get the client back in the community if he can handle it."

Not everyone was convinced. Doubters included some of Pineland's doctors and other staff members, union officials, and parents. "Pineland Center's new approach causes an uproar," said a headline in Augusta's *Kennebec Journal*. Although some were satisfied with and excited by the changes, the discontent of others continued to build, and spring 1975 found groups of parents and union members picketing together outside Pineland's administrative building to protest policies and demand a new legislative investigation.

By this point, major changes had occurred in Augusta. Kearns had resigned his commissioner's job as the administration of Governor Kenneth Curtis left office. James B. Longley became the new governor, and Dr. John Rosser the new commissioner. Longley visited Pineland while Wurtz was still there, and the superintendent used the visit to protest the governor's refusal to fill vacancies left by a 50

What William F. Kearns Jr. has done in his four years as commissioner is to bring about change in an agency which provides services to minds and bodies, ministering to psyches and souls.

Many of the changes grate harshly against both the puritan ethic and the traditional concept of institutionalization held by some Maine legislators and departmental employees. They have, consequently, placed Commissioner Kearns in the type of hotseat formerly reserved primarily for commissioners of economic development.

Fortunately for Kearns, his legislative critics are neither as powerful nor as influential as they may themselves believe or as their trumpeting criticisms in the press would lead the public to conclude they are.

—*Donald C. Hansen in* Maine Sunday Telegram, *May 6, 1973*

percent turnover in psychiatric aides. The refusal would destroy unitization, Wurtz believed, but the governor stood firm. Not long after that, the new team decided that it wanted fresh leadership in Pineland, and Wurtz resigned his post, effective at the end of June 1975.

Continuing Movement Toward Deinstitutionalization

The concerns of many Pineland critics intensified in the 1970s in response to a report that the whole institution might close. Not so, said Superintendent Wurtz and Commissioner Kearns in 1973, Director Anderson in 1974, and Commissioner Rosser in 1975. But deinstitutionalization was continuing, and Pineland's population was decreasing. By March 1975 the patient population was just 493—down to 60 percent of its 1969 level. Attempts to move more residents into the community continued to be strong. Regional officials from Augusta were actively working to help identify and develop community nursing homes, boarding facilities, and foster homes that could accept more Pineland clients.

Deinstitutionalization was inappropriate for many, critics contended, in part because Maine had failed to do the comprehensive planning necessary to create the community care envisioned by federal legislation in the early 1960s. In 1975, the American Federation of State, County and Municipal Employees issued a thirty-five-page report giving eighteen examples of failed community placements from the state's three mental institutions. The report concluded:

> *In summary, the deinstitutionalization policy seems to have been prompted more by political and economic considerations than by the devel-*

opment of a planned treatment strategy for the chronic mentally ill or mentally retarded citizens in this state. The movement of patients from the public institutions to the private boarding and nursing care industry is a means of transferring financial responsibility for health care from the state to the federal government, without enhancing health services in the process.

There could be problems, agreed proponents of deinstitutionalization. But the community could and would develop the facilities needed to handle this new, more effective and humane approach. Moreover, the change would help those remaining at Pineland, Wurtz argued. The reduction in population meant that there were more employees than residents at the center, he said as he prepared to leave office. The staff could now give its attention to the most challenging cases. "We're doing training now with severely and profoundly retarded. This was unheard of five or ten years ago."

Who's Minding the Store?

Changes in administrators responsible for Pineland continued a pattern identified by the *Maine Sunday Telegram* of June 10, 1973. At that point, nine men had

> . . . Carroll lives a quiet life reading and taking care of his pet chickens.
>
> He spoke slowly in Yankee style, much like Mr. Little [owner of the home where he lived]. Carroll fondly recalled his [Pownal State School] days and seemed to feel it was his real home. Like Ethel Beecher, he was often sorry he ever left. Carroll seems to be very alert and to be of at least average intelligence. His disposition is placid. He is fond of the Littles, and Mr. Little seemed very fond of him. The latter appears to treat him with respect, and seemed quite in awe of "all his reading."
>
> Carroll asked about the location of a patient whom he took care of at PSS. He said he would like to write to him or, if possible, see him. He also recalled how he used to "write letters for everyone on Sundays."
>
> *—An interview reported in John L. Hoffman's study of former Pineland residents, published in 1969. Names were changed for the report. Carroll had entered Pownal State School in 1933 at age forty-three and stayed for twenty-five years. He was committed by town officials after his father's death because of his physical disability and despite his apparently normal intelligence.*

The Committee met with Commissioner Kearns during the course of its study to elicit from him the facts needed to complete its investigation. The Commissioner told the Committee that he wished that they would "keep their noses out of his business" and further indicated that "the Legislature has no right to interfere with the administrative and executive policies."

—*State of Maine Health and Institutional Services Committee, "Report on Study of the Department of Mental Health and Corrections," February 1973*

recently been "fired, retired or transferred to another line of work" from senior positions in the seven institutions supervised by the Department of Mental Health and Corrections. The pattern was national in scope, Wurtz told the *Kennebec Journal* at the time of his own departure. "What's happening in Maine is true in every state that is making changes. Superintendencies and bureau director jobs are turning over quite rapidly."

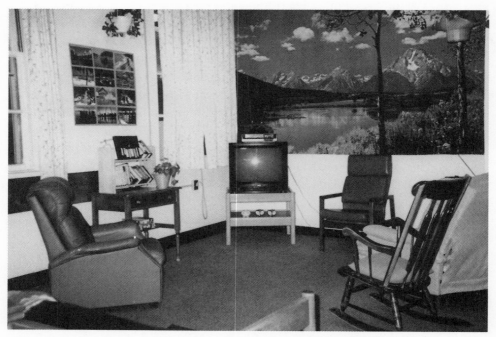

Cumberland Hall living room (courtesy of the New Gloucester Historical Society)

Actually, the pace of change would soon pick up at Pineland. Looking back from 1983, John L. Hoffman, Pineland's social research scientist, summarized the period:

The earlier part of the seventies was marked by a degree of turmoil at Pineland. Certain forces saw a need for the total elimination of the facility, since they defined any "institution" per se as evil. Other forces sought Pineland's limited continuation with redefined purposes and internal improvements. The facility itself was the battleground for these conflicting elements. During most of this decade the stability that comes from continuous personal direction was lacking. While there had been only five different Superintendents in the 63 year period from 1908 to 1971, there were ten changes from 1971 to 1979 of Superintendents or Acting Superintendents.

Many other people also earnestly sought to help shape Pineland's destiny. They included members of the unions at the school; parents around the state; legislators, department administrators, and various governors in Augusta; and journal-

---

POWNAL, Maine—Ed Degerstrom is middle-aged and retarded, and he has spent much of his life at the Pineland Hospital and Training Center propped up in a reclining chair because his limbs are too twisted to support him.

But since early this year Degerstrom has been able to sit up straight; not because of any treatment breakthrough, but because somebody built him a chair.

The somebody is Wendell Strong, a carpenter at Pineland for 16 years.

Degerstrom's chair is a masterpiece of simplicity and recycled parts. Strong stripped a wheelchair to its frame, then built it up again with a new seat, back, footrest and tray, all done to Degerstrom's measurements. . . .

Each patient at Pineland has a special need. Some need foot splints and braces, others need "crutches" to hold them upright in the chair. A girl with a back deformity has a chair with part of the back support cut out and padded to conform to her body.

For Strong it's demanding work that he likes.

"I don't look at it as a pain," he said. "Before, I was always just repairing something. There was nothing gained. I feel like I'm really doing something for the first time since I've been here."

—Boston Globe, *August 19, 1973*

> Camp Tall Pines is a summer day camp owned and maintained by the Volunteers of Pineland, Inc., for the express purpose of providing a wholesome camping and outdoor recreation program for the entire population of Pineland Hospital and Training Center. In four short years it has become one of the most innovative, progressive and well staffed camping facilities for the retarded in the State of Maine. A twenty-eight foot pontoon raft was purchased by the Volunteers of Pineland, Inc. through the strong efforts of the Lewiston-Auburn Kiwanis Club. This boat now makes it possible for the profoundly and severely retarded as well as the multiply handicapped to enjoy boat rides on Lower Range Pond. Never have so many of Pineland residents participated in a complete program of nature crafts, camping skills, team sports, boating, swimming, cooking, overnight camping, hiking and music as in the summer of 1971 [when total summer attendance over 13 weeks was 3,040, and when 32 volunteers gave a total of 348 hours].
> —*Pineland Hospital and Training Center annual report, June 30, 1972*

ists from near and far. With all these sometimes competing forces at work, it might have seemed unlikely that any new force would enter the scene and assume a controlling role affecting all the others, but that is just what occurred.

The Court

The new player was the United States District Court in Portland, invited to the fray by various parties, including people who worked at the school. One deeply involved person was Allison Anspach, a young woman hired in 1974 by the commissioner of the Department of Mental Health and Corrections to represent and advocate for the residents of Pineland. She worked at the institution, though not directly for it. In May 1975, the *Lewiston Sun Journal* introduced her to its readers:

> *"I have a narrow, consumer-oriented perspective," she explained, "all from the point of view of the residents."*
>
> *The position is now about a year old. As former Superintendent Conrad Wurtz described it, the function is to ask whether Pineland is "providing for the human and civil rights of our clients."*
>
> *"Basically the retarded person has the same rights as any individual," said Ms. Anspach.*
>
> *"For a minor, those include the rights to adequate care and protection, and to a public education. For all residents, it includes the right to keep*

their liberty or property, and not be deprived of that unless by due process of the law."

Ensuring the rights of the retarded had gained national favor in the years since Pearl Buck wrote of her daughter's experiences and since the federal government and other institutions began extensive new efforts to assist and protect the disabled. But achieving the goal at an aging, underfunded, and understaffed institution such as Pineland would not be easy, no matter how many people applauded the general idea. Niedorf was not the only senior administrator who thought court action might be necessary to straighten things out. Others included Wurtz, who later remembered quietly looking the other way while Ansbach and others prepared to sue his organization and its leaders.

The effort was already under way in May 1975, according to the *Sun Journal* report, which said, "Pine Tree Legal Assistance is currently planning, with the assistance of Ms. Anspach and others such as the Maine Association for Retarded Citizens, a class action right to treatment suit against the institution, claiming residents are not being offered adequate care."

This was, after all, a period of national court activism. Judges across the country had begun issuing opinions that favored the disadvantaged and forced states and communities to honor the rights of all. Leading the way was Judge Frank M. Johnson, Jr., who sat on the federal bench in Montgomery, Alabama. Johnson had won fame in the 1950s and 1960s for civil rights rulings involving famous protestors such as Rosa Parks and Martin Luther King, Jr. Early in the 1970s, Johnson declared Alabama's state mental hospitals to be "human warehouses" and issued

Skip's principal duty as advocate at Pineland is to serve as a grievance-response mechanism for the clients of Pineland Center. He depends upon staff for input to keep informed of problems affecting our clients. He asks that anyone knowing about or having seen any client denied their rights (including basic civil rights, medical care, including dental care; freedom from abuse; the least restrictive methods of care and treatment; pay for work performed; adequate care, including proper clothing, hygiene supplies, warmth, food, proper sanitation, etc.; treatment, including education, training, recreation, P.T., O.T., Speech and Hearing therapy, psychological counseling, etc.; and the right to individual dignity); please contact him.
—Pineland Observer, *July-August 1977, describing the work of Carroll M. "Skip" Macgowan, a new resident advocate*

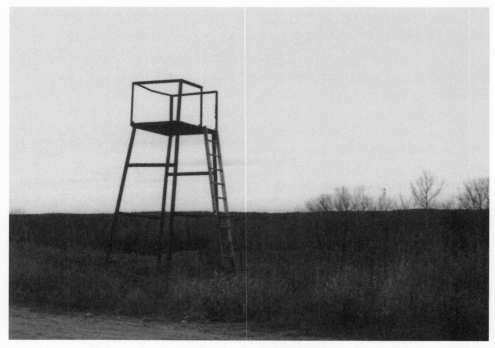

Observation post for spotting wandering residents, at Valley Farm (courtesy of Elaine Gallant)

far-reaching orders establishing the right of patients to receive adequate care. He stated in detail what Alabama had to do for them. News of his decision would encourage fresh legal initiatives in many other states, including Maine. These initiatives would also produce some interesting results, setting standards for care and defining fair treatment for residents—requiring, for example, just payment for any work performed by residents at places such as Pineland.

In fact, Pine Tree Legal Assistance itself was a product of the new national interest in helping the disadvantaged. It had been funded with the help of federal monies in 1966 as a nonprofit corporation to provide legal assistance to low-income Maine residents. Its director-attorney in the early 1970s was Neville Woodruff, a near neighbor of Pineland. Woodruff had already assigned himself as the lawyer to fulfill a Pine Tree contract with Maine to advocate for retarded people around the state. Now an intense spring investigation had convinced him, Ansbach, and others that a major class action suit was the only way to protect the rights of 500 residents at Pineland as well as 500 Pineland clients—the term used for previous residents living outside the institution.

Pine Tree filed suit on July 3, 1975, basing its case on an eighteen-page complaint naming Martti Wuori and six other residents as plaintiffs, and acting super-

Thank god you're here! I haven't had a break yet. Here—take this mop and bucket. And don't turn your back!

> —*An aide in Yarmouth Hall greeting Skip Macgowan on the day in 1975 he visited Pineland to check on job possibilities. An administrator had directed him to Yarmouth, where he stayed during the attendant's break and watched forty-nine men, "the three wearing johnnies the most dressed of them all." Though tempted to flee Pineland forever, Macgowan took a job teaching "older active boys—a euphemism for aggressive." He kept that job for fourteen months before becoming an advocate.*

intendent Margaret Bruns along with fourteen other officials at Pineland and in Augusta as defendants.

The plaintiffs, said the complaint, "have hoped to have the needs for safe and healthful care met and they have hoped to receive the education and training which would enable them so far as possible to lead normal lives." But the state was failing them.

> *Although Pineland Center has been in the throes of change for at least the last several years, their hopes are no closer to being realized.*
>
> *Instead, acute boredom, physical deterioration, social regression, psychological debilitation, severe depression and low morale predominate.*

Detailed allegations spoke of "rooms that smelled of urine and feces," of dental care denied, of a laundry worker fired after a court ruling that said he should be paid, of curtainless showers and inadequate toilet supplies, of school training limited to five hours a week. More generally, said the complaint:

> *Because the staff is not large enough, many must work overtime and consequently nerves are frayed and performance is poor. Little provision is made for staff training and upgrading of skills.*
>
> *[Plaintiffs] are denied their rights to a safe and healthful environment and to that kind of care, education and treatment reasonably calculated to bring about their improvement and normalization in violation of the due process clause of the Fourteenth Amendment.*

There were a lot of good workers at Pineland and a lot of good things happened there. The staff weren't bad people, but some bad things happened. Some of the kids had bad stories about what "daddy" or "mumma" did to them. That's what they called the people who took care of them.

—*Mickey Boutelier, director of Maine Special Olympics, looking back in the year 2000 on his long involvement with Pineland*

Keeping plaintiffs at Pineland against their will, purportedly to meet their needs for habilitation, but under the conditions alleged here, amounts to cruel and unusual punishment prohibited by the Eighth Amendment . . .

Only the most intensive efforts by defendants directed toward plaintiffs' complete habilitation can begin to undo the consequences of past neglect.

Money damages cannot adequately compensate them for the care and treatment defendants have denied plaintiffs while at Pineland.

With the filing of these words, Pineland began another round of change, a round that would do much to determine its ultimate fate.

Staying Out of Court

The class action suit would never go to trial. Officials in Augusta initially promised to contest the charges of the suit, and the state apparently at first intended to do real battle. News reports quite consistently spoke of the suit in terms of a two-sided struggle. But defendants had only to glance around to recognize their time as an era of court activism when unprecedented federal decisions had already forced significant social change. It was crystal clear that a trial might well result in forced change. Besides, some of the defendants supported that change; they very much wanted Pineland to do more for its residents. "This was a 'sue me please' lawsuit," said Jeffrey Lee, remembering back from the year 2000. Lee was a lawyer who joined Pineland's staff as a resident advocate in 1979 and later became the center's acting superintendent. "Not everybody wanted change but a lot of them did. And they could see what was happening in similar lawsuits around the country."

Also looking back from the year 2000, Woodruff recalled that he had met more resistance in Augusta than on the grounds of Pineland. Not everybody on the campus was happy when he appeared on his frequent visits. He deeply irritated some employees with his endless digging into records but greatly impressed others as he

> I always thought of them as kids. I had to. If any man on the outside ever did to me what some of them did, he'd have been a blood splat on the wall.
> —*Nancy L. Wilcox, Pineland secretary, looking back from the year 2000*

visited with residents and staff. In general, he concluded later, "the reception to the suit was good from the superintendent on down." Not everybody agreed with every complaint, of course, but several superintendents and other employees at lower levels were very cooperative. Some testified frankly that Pineland as then operating simply could not provide all the services its residents required. Plaintiffs also drew considerable support from a study that Pineland researcher John L. Hoffman had done into the fate of 1,800 former residents released during the Bowman years. "Jack had a federal grant for about a year to find these people," according to Woodruff. His report was "really pretty exciting reading," because it showed that "a huge portion" of them had been "totally integrated into the community. Here was the proof that Pineland's size was ridiculous."

With the approval and direction of Judge Edward T. Gignoux, attorneys for the two sides began seriously negotiating a settlement. The state also began to act, and Attorney General Joseph E. Brennan directed an investigation that supported complaints about Pineland:

> *Significantly it has been determined that the majority of residents are housed in relatively sterile, barracklike housing rather than in a homelike environment consistent with the goal of returning each resident to his home.*
>
> *Large numbers of residents who need speech and hearing therapy do not receive it due to lack of resources.*
>
> *Each resident between the ages of 5 and 20 does not receive the schooling guaranteed him.*
>
> *Large numbers of residents in need of physical therapy do not receive such therapy due to lack of resources.*
>
> *Large numbers of residents lacking the skills necessary to clothe, bathe, feed and groom themselves are not provided with the occupational therapy necessary to acquire these skills due to lack of resources.*

With this emerging support for change, Governor James B. Longley and the legislature moved in April 1976 to provide almost $1 million in new money to Pineland. Conditions improved to the point of winning fresh approval from the Joint Commission on Accreditation of Hospitals, which had found the school below

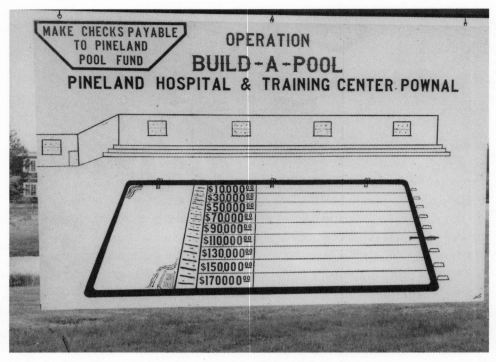

A fund-raising sign on campus (courtesy of the Maine State Archives)

its standards after an inspection in 1974. That sounded promising for residents of the school, Woodruff told reporters. But what about clients whom Pineland had placed in other facilities? They were also plaintiffs in the case. Negotiations continued.

There were positive physical improvements, too. On June 25, 1976, the governor's wife and David Cook, a Pineland resident, posed together with a shovel used in the ceremonial groundbreaking for a new therapeutic swimming pool that Pineland had wanted for twenty-five years. The state had kicked in $50,000, the Pineland Parents and Friends had provided $16,000, and the Joseph P. Kennedy, Jr., Foundation had given $1,000 more. But the largest share, more than $50,000, came from Maine union members. The AFL-CIO had spent six years raising the money, getting $12,000 of it at a 1975 fund-raiser at which President Gerald R. Ford appeared (and donated $20). Members of the U.S. Naval Reserves had kept costs down by preparing a site next to the Soucy gym. The new facility would be good for residents, but it could not by itself answer plaintiff complaints, and negotiations went on.

> The Legislature finds and declares that the rights of mentally retarded persons can be protected best under a system of care which operates according to the principles of normalization. . . . "Normalization principle" means the principle of letting the mentally retarded persons obtain an existence as close to normal as possible and making available to them patterns and conditions of everyday life which are as close as possible to the norms and patterns of the mainstream of society.
> — *"An Act to Establish a Bill of Rights for Mentally Retarded Persons" in Maine, 1977*

A year later the legislature passed and the governor signed an act establishing a bill of rights for mentally retarded persons, a bill subscribing to the "principles of normalization," calling for further development of community-based services, requiring pay for resident labor, and promising to help retarded citizens lead independent and productive lives. This too was welcomed by critics of Pineland, but it was not enough to end their concern, and they refused to accept it as the total solution that some defendants said it was. Again negotiations continued, but now with state officials—in the words of Woodruff—becoming increasingly serious about putting together "something that would really hold water."

Pine Tree at this point was being assisted by lawyers from the Mental Health Law Project of Washington, D.C. Leading players on the state's side included George A. Zitnay, Pineland's superintendent for a year before he moved on to Augusta as Mental Health and Corrections commissioner in October 1975, and Kevin Concannon, director of the Bureau of Mental Retardation.

Finally, on July 14, 1978, three years after the process had started, Judge Gignoux signed a consent decree that plaintiffs and defendants alike called a "landmark." It "goes further or is more clear than any other decree that has been entered anywhere in the country," Woodruff told reporters. "Even more dramatic is that for the first time the standards applicable to institutionalized persons are also applicable to persons residing in the community."

The decree directed Pineland to continue placing residents into the community. The resident population, at 500 when the suit was filed and at 450 when it was settled, must drop to 350 within two years. And care of the retarded both inside and outside the institution must change dramatically in many directions.

Appendix A of the decree presented forty-six pages of Pineland Program Standards, covering everything from walls around toilets to diet, from use of consultants to use of restraint chairs, from schooling to grooming. Care would be indi-

> One time two of us had to drive over to Lewiston to pick up a kid who had run away. We went to the police station and they had some drunk in there sleeping it off. The kid was really in the county jail, but they didn't know that. So they went and woke the drunk guy up. He was still drunker than hell and he looked up at us and saw us all dressed in white. "Not me," he said. "Not me," over and over. You should have seen him. His mother must have told him that the men in white were going to come get him if he kept on drinking.
>
> —*Conrad Lausier, ambulance driver, looking back from the year 2000*

vidualized by teams of staff members, and a Prescriptive Program Plan (PPP) would be developed for each resident. Said a paragraph from the program standards:

> *Each resident shall receive assistance in learning normal grooming and personal hygiene practices. Individual toilet articles shall be available to each resident unless contradicted by the resident's PPP. Residents shall receive a bath or shower at least every other day. Hair styling and finger and toe nail cutting shall be regularly scheduled for all residents.*

Appendix B of the settlement set similar standards for Pineland clients living outside the institution. These were a source of special pride for Woodruff. "I think I deserve credit for that," he said. "Our case for community standards was a little thin, but we managed to hold everything together until the end. We showed you couldn't just release people into the community without support services."

Beyond the Settlement

It would be difficult to overstate the impact of the Martti Wuori case on Pineland. Although there was a settlement, it did not bring settled conditions to the institution. The consent decree covered many different facets of Pineland's operation, affecting almost everything and everybody there. Numerous staff members would spend the next several years working toward a state of full compliance, sometimes at a frantic pace and always with the sense of being watched by David D. Gregory, special master for the United States District Court, the man appointed by Judge Gignoux to ensure compliance with the decree.

Encouraging press reports began to appear almost as soon as the suit was settled. "Court-Ordered Changes Already Dramatic Ones," proclaimed the *Press Herald* on August 22, 1978, above an article that read in part:

Pineland Center is shedding its skin.

The state's largest institution for the mentally handicapped is in the midst of a court-ordered metamorphosis—no longer what it was, not yet what it will become. . . .

Buildings too run-down to be renovated have been vacated. Large open wards that once housed dozens of persons in cramped quarters have been converted into smaller more private units. Doors are being installed on the toilets, curtains are being put up on the walls; rugs, personal wardrobes and posters are being used to give the rooms a touch of individualism.

But the change at Pineland is not merely a physical transformation.

These two act like a couple of sisters together. Mavis [a former Pineland resident] is a sweet, gentle woman who needs and works at keeping harmony within the home. Mrs. T. [with whom she boards] admits that she gets cross sometimes and when this happens, Mavis inevitably will ask if she is out of cigarettes, and if so, there is some haste to see that she is supplied with these adult pacifiers. Mrs. T. becomes so amused at this device that it probably serves its purpose very well.

Mavis . . . appears to be in good health. Their diet seems rather questionable as both are too stout and Mrs. T., who does all the cooking, will sometimes whip up a pie which goes for the entire meal and is apparently devoured at one sitting. Both women chuckle over this like a couple of kids. The apartment, one-half of a duplex, is very neat, cheerful, and allows for plenty of room for them both. Mrs. T. may be a little on the fatalistic side, but this seems like a reasonably serene, pleasant situation for our ex-pt.

> *—An interview reported in John L. Hoffman's study of former Pineland residents, published in 1969. Names were changed for the report. Mavis had entered the Maine School for Feeble-Minded (MSFM) in 1910 at age nine and stayed until 1960. "The mother was probably mentally very limited," according to the interview notes, "and an eccentric and mean-spirited stepfather had Mavis placed in the City Poor Farm, which in turn sent her to MSFM. Rather curiously, the stepfather spent the rest of his life trying to get Mavis back again, but without success."*

Residents who for years did little more than stare at four walls and a ceiling are now engaged in programmed activity aimed at helping them achieve a normal lifestyle. The use of both physical and chemical restraints has been cut back dramatically. Ninety of the institution's 440 residents are targeted for placement in a community-based residential facility within the next two years.

State officials were encouraging, too. News reports in January 1979 said that Director Concannon at the Bureau of Mental Retardation was "delighted" with the Pineland changes.

Photographs found in the archives today support the optimism of the period; they depict an increasing range of often engaging resident activities—creating with finger paints, playing with parachutes in the gym, building ice sculptures, and joining in organized sports.

But tensions mounted in early 1979 as the time approached for a hearing about Pineland's progress in achieving compliance. In March, Charlene Kinnelly, acting superintendent, wrote a memo alerting the staff to possible visits by Neville Woodruff and directing that any conversations with him be reported to her. "This hearing is extremely serious and I do not wish to have any breakdowns in communication," she said.

Trouble was brewing all right, but it was to come from the special master. Gregory failed to share Concannon's delight in Pineland's development. In fact, he said in a report dated March 19, Concannon himself was about the only official involved who deserved praise for the limited progress made. "The lion's share of praise for those accomplishments which have occurred belongs to the Director of the Bureau of Mental Retardation," Gregory wrote. "He has been tireless in his efforts to develop new community residences and programs and to spread the message of the court's decree throughout the State."

Pineland Center, on the other hand, "displays a worshipful devotion to foolish, cumbersome, convoluted Pineland procedures. With exceptions, it avoids imaginative problem solving and excels in producing reasons why things cannot be done."

Looking back from the twenty-first century, Concannon rejected parts of Gregory's assessment. The problem was that the staff had not yet been brought on board, he said. Will Burrow, the superintendent involved in helping negotiate the settlement, had left, and others still had to figure out what it was all about. Gregory had "a great passion" for getting things done immediately, but there was a lot to do and it couldn't happen all at once.

Gregory's dissatisfaction continued through the next several months, and in November it hit the press through a blistering report submitted to the federal court.

A number of our dischargees have attained an "ideal" level of performance that combines economic independence with a mature and cooperative social self-sufficiency that one might expect to find in responsible members of society at large.

—*John L. Hoffman's study of former Pineland residents, published in 1969*

"Pineland Center is not complying with the order of the court," he said. "Noncompliance is substantial and continuing. In no major area is Pineland Center meeting the court decree."

State officials fought back. "The staff has been fantastic," said George A. Zitnay, who had run into political problems as commissioner of Mental Health and Corrections, then returned in October for a second stint as Pineland's superintendent. "I'm extremely disappointed with his statement," said Michael R. Petit, commissioner of the Department of Human Services. "I don't know what the report is based on but it's not an accurate assessment."

A new attorney general, Richard S. Cohen, responded to Gregory in a thirteen-page report to Judge Gignoux. He offered a long list of improvements made at Pineland, from increasing the staff size to establishing eight new program centers, and from establishing a beauty salon to providing more bathroom privacy. The court master's attitudes raised "a serious question" about his "ability to continue serving," said Cohen. Gregory had "failed to follow the court order to develop an evaluation system to measure the degree of compliance, and instead has used the information gathered for him as an argument to close Pineland, which neither the court, nor the state had contemplated."

Indeed, Gregory had expressed a strong distrust of institutions. "Every single task undertaken in a custodial institution is more difficult and more expensive and produces worse results than in a more normal environment," he said in his report. "The simplest prescriptions of the court's decree—provide normal clothing, provide normal meals, provide a warm homelike environment, provide privacy, dignity and comfort—cannot be met by a custodial institution. They are not being met at Pineland."

Soon parents and the public were joining the debate. The state's reaction to the court master was a "cop-out," said the mother of a mentally handicapped boy in a letter to the *Press Herald* of January 14, 1980. "The stigma of Pineland's name and its rurally isolated area will last far longer than the state has money to keep it in operation according to the court decree's orders."

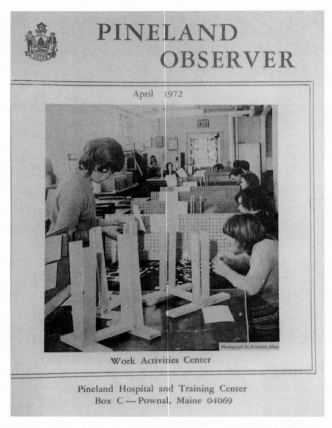

Pineland Observer, *April 1972 (courtesy of the New Gloucester Historical Society)*

"As parents of a 22-year-old retarded daughter who has been in Pineland Center for one year we can see satisfactory results already," said another letter in the same paper. "She seems happy, has put on needed weight and has a more relaxed appearance."

And so the Pineland decade closed with as much disagreement as had clouded its beginning. But beneath the clouds was a dramatically changed institution. The Pineland of the early 1980s would be markedly different from the Pineland of the early 1970s.

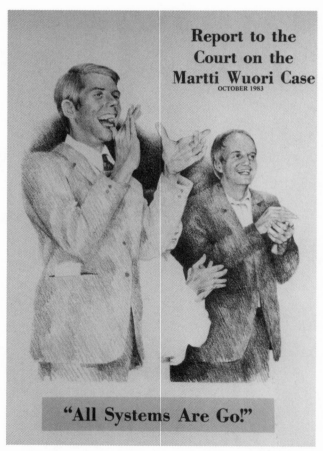

A report to the court (courtesy of the New Gloucester Historical Society)

Ascent and Decline: The 1980s

"Pineland has new name, fresh outlook," said a *Portland Press Herald* headline on May 12, 1980. The new name was Pineland: A Comprehensive Center for the Developmentally Disabled. The new outlook was based in progress toward the goals established by the consent decree: renovating buildings, increasing staff size, decreasing resident numbers, regulating patient restraints and medications, and providing carefully programmed activities for each resident every day.

The innovations were evident in Doris Anderson Hospital, said the report:

> *Two years ago most of the young men living at Doris Anderson had serious behavior problems. They destroyed much of the new furniture, raced up and down the hallways and spent their time rocking to and fro in chairs in the recreation room. The bedroom doors had to be locked to keep residents from tearing apart the contents.*
>
> *Last week it was quieter. The doors were no longer locked. The rooms didn't resemble prison cells. Most residents were out. The building has been remodeled.*
>
> *And it is now coed.*

Not that everything was perfect. Two months after that article appeared, the *Press Herald*'s sister publication, the *Evening Express*, offered a headline with quite a different spirit: "Controversies still rage over conditions at Pineland Center." All parties agreed that Pineland had moved far beyond the snake pit era of the 1960s, but there were many doubts about its abilities to achieve all of the decree's objectives.

159

CHANGING PINES
Strangely, I felt the room empty.
Plain walls, stark corners,
blinding lights and terrible smells,
memories of years ago.
People packed in a small space.
No time for anyone of them,
working hard, but they get little comfort.
I shake my head out of the daydream.
Look around and see the room's filled
with John watching a movie,
pretty posters, plants and Teddy Bears
More time for special things.
I feel a great weight taken off
and believe they feel it too.

—*Elaine Gallant, on returning to Pineland in the
late 1970s and seeing the changes made during a
break of a few years*

Some of the goals, in fact, seemed contradictory and impossible. The decree required Pineland to treat each resident for six hours a day, Superintendent George Zitnay told reporters. But it also said that patients could not be forced to accept training, so Pineland could not always comply with the ruling. Such loopholes needed court attention, he said.

The court master remained highly skeptical of Pineland's chances. "All is not well," said Pinky Karwowski, president of Pineland Parents and Friends, speaking through the *Observer* early in 1980.

We can't praise too highly all the wonderful people we have met and dealt with at Pineland Center. Sidney John loved them all, and they him. We will go far and wide to sing the Praises of Pineland.

—*Testimony from the parents of a resident who died
at Cumberland Hall in 1978*

There looms on the horizon a dark cloud, in the form of the recent report of the court, that may dampen the spirits of those providing the care of our loved ones.

It would be my sincerest new year goal that together, we accept the Court Master's report as a challenge and use it as a tool by which we can further enrich the lives of our mentally handicapped citizens.

The chances of that happening were better than they seemed to many. Doubts and problems surely remained, but a progressive momentum had been achieved.

1. The trainer should check the toothbrush to see if it is in good condition with no bristles missing. If the resident is capable of doing this he should be taught to check his own brush. Now the resident should learn to apply toothpaste to his brush. If the resident does not have his own toothpaste he should learn to apply the toothpaste to a piece of paper towel then apply it to the brush. (If this is impractical the trainer will prepare the toothpaste on the paper towel before the training session.) This will eliminate the chance of cross contamination.

   Cue words: 1. "Check your brush." OPTIONAL.

   2. "Put toothpaste on your brush." OPTIONAL.

   3. "Put the cap back on the toothpaste." OPTIONAL

2. Teach the resident to put the toothbrush to the outside back and brush the upper and lower teeth on one side of his mouth. Then have him repeat this on the other side of his mouth.

   Cue words: 1. "Put the toothbrush to the back of your mouth."

   2. "Now brush your teeth."

   3. "Now do the other side."

Give the resident as much assistance as he needs at first, gradually fading it out. Teach the resident to clear his mouth if necessary.

   4. "Spit."

—From volume 2 of the Maine Bureau of Mental Retardation's program guide for Pineland Center, dated 1975, prepared under grants and carrying the names of Albert Anderson, Jr., Ph.D., director of the bureau, and Conrad R. Wurtz, Ph.D., Pineland's superintendent. This segment represents a third of a page from a four-page section on brushing teeth.

Forces of Continuing Change

Contemporary attitudes toward retardation, new groups concerned with place and program, institutional self-interest, and the dedication of many administrators and staff members all helped sustain Pineland's forward movement.

"Deinstitutionalization" and "normalization" continued to be effective buzzwords not just at Pineland but at similar institutions around the country, and not just in the field of retardation but in the world of mental illness as well. National trends were very clear. As James W. Trent, Jr., put it in *Inventing the Feeble Mind*:

> *In this confluence—one, of state officials eager to shift responsibilities for services to the federal level; two, of civil libertarians ready to close inhumane institutions and segregated special classes; and three, of a vision of normalization that provided a rationale and method for opening communities to disabled people—the deinstitutionalization of mentally retarded people from public facilities was rapid and continuous.*

At Pineland, the number of residents had decreased to 370 by May 1980, and staffers were working hard to decrease it further—despite some trepidation on the part of families and residents. Zitnay offered this explanation in the *Observer* for the winter of 1982–83:

> *It is the role of the Bureau and Pineland to return the residents as close as possible to their family and into an environment that will help them to continue to grow. . . . For some parents . . . this is a hard decision because they are comfortable and familiar with Pineland and the Pineland Center Staff. For some residents of Pineland it is extremely difficult because Pineland has become their home.*

Federal legislation and funds now supported intermediate care facilities that provided alternatives to larger institutions. Some of these were established in communities beyond Pineland and some at the center itself. The Intermediate Care–Mentally Retarded (ICF/MR) units had to meet a separate set of federal standards. Those at Pineland, said *The Maine Paper*, had "the appearance of modern, well-equipped nursing homes" and cared for residents unable to function in the apartment settings found elsewhere on the grounds.

At Pineland, too, new watchdog and support groups were present and would work throughout the 1980s to ensure the implementation and continuing enforcement of the court order. One was the Consumer Advisory Board established by the decree. It had nine members appointed by the commissioner of the Department of Mental Health and Corrections, among them parents or relatives of residents, residents or former residents, Pineland's resident advocate and chaplain, and com-

> Monday, January 4, 1982
> Well what an exciting evening!
> Have been on auxiliary power since approx 1:15 p.m. - All units notified.
> Things going smoothly until about 5:15 p.m. when we blew a big - big fuse - lost everything, phones, power, courage.
> Rain, rain and tons of slush -
>
> —*Shift supervisor's log*

munity leaders. Its broad duties, said the *Observer*, "include the evaluation of alleged dehumanizing practices at Pineland Center, the promotion of the normalization of the institution, and the examination of violations of individual rights." The board was charged as well with finding "correspondents," or volunteer supporters for all residents within Pineland and all clients now living outside who lacked legal guardians, parents, or other family members who would represent them to the board.

A five-person Board of Visitors also helped monitor progress under the consent decree. In 1985 the board began holding Pineland hearings to conduct "a searching review of progress made and that which remains to be accomplished on behalf of mentally retarded citizens," in the words of its chair, William Flahive, dean of Adult and Continuing Education at the Southern Maine Vocational-Technical Institute.

Residents—now often referred to by the *Observer* as "men and women" instead of "boys and girls"—had their own Resident Council, formed in 1978 and led by Pineland's resident advocate and chaplain.

Cheryl E. Fortier, a resident advocate from 1977 to 1980 and again beginning in 1990, later remembered the council as helpful but somewhat recreational in tone. "It wasn't like people were going to let the council run the place," she said. Still, members of the council could be helpful. "For example, you could ask people who lived here what they thought about being called 'residents.'" And what did they think? "They didn't like that at all. They didn't want to be called anything that set them apart. They wanted to be called 'people.' So I often called them 'the people who live here,' and I called the staff 'the people who work here.'"

Nancy L. Thomas, an advocate in the 1980s, later agreed that although residents could speak out through advocates and occasional committees and groups, theirs was not a controlling voice. "There was no real formal way for them to have an impact on policy. By then, a lot of the higher functioning residents had already left. So any impact they had was on a case by case basis."

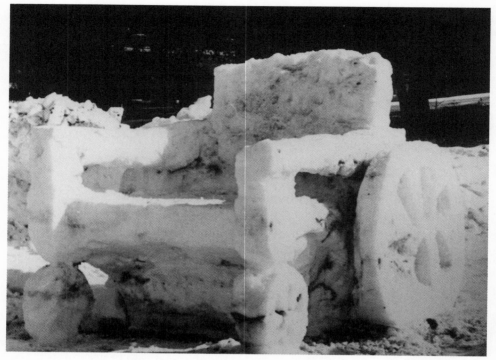

Sculpted ice chair (courtesy of the New Gloucester Historical Society)

The advocates also remained a strong force for change. One of them was Carroll M. "Skip" Macgowan, who had come to Pineland as a teacher in 1975 and later replaced Allison Anspach as advocate. Like Anspach, he was located in but independent of the institution, and could work to help residents secure their rights and full support in areas ranging from hygiene to dignity, from clothing to work. His surveillance was careful and intense; years later he recalled moving around the Pineland grounds with the department's chief advocate from Augusta. "We would visit any building at any time, day or night, to see what was going on."

Macgowan was active beyond the grounds as well; in the early 1980s he became instrumental in securing passage of a new sterilization law, which was passed partly

> November 29, 1983
> E_S_ choked on food at noon meal today. It required much attention to revive him. R_F_, nurses, physicians, all responded very quickly.
> —*Shift supervisor's log*

> We got permission to plant a small garden and we were looking forward to all the goodies we could have from our garden. We just needed to have it turned over and then we could begin.
>
> June told us all we could grow was rocks! We couldn't find anything equipment wise to turn the ground over—there really were all rocks. What a disappointment.
>
> —Pineland Observer *report on a project at Bliss Hall, summer 1980*

to reinforce the rights of people with retardation. Through the years, 206 recorded sterilizations had been performed on Maine retarded people, but none had been done since 1969, when the involuntary sterilization of a nineteen-year-old girl from Guilford resulted in court action. The new law was required partly to protect the retarded from sterilization and partly to ensure their rights to sterilization in a time when such voluntary surgical birth control was increasingly favored by the general population.

The state and Pineland could ill afford failure, which could have smeared very dark blots on individual career records and led to court takeover of the center. Expenses were already soaring; by 1980 the cost of running Pineland was more than twice the $4.7 million budgeted in 1970. Expenses were sure to go higher still if the court took charge. "The worst thing that could happen would be for the court to take over the operation itself," Senator David G. Huber, a Republican from Falmouth, told a reporter. "They'd just go ahead and make the changes and bill us for the total cost." So there was impetus for movement from above, impetus reflected in Augusta by a change in the department responsible for Pineland. In 1981 the Department of Mental Health and Corrections became the Department of Mental Health and Mental Retardation; the Department of Corrections became a separate entity.

Many Pineland employees needed little pressure from Augusta to implement new ideas. Of course there were pockets of resistance—those who liked the old ways, those more comfortable with inertia than motion. But others were delighted with the court's ruling and eager to improve resident care. Among these was Mary Crichton, who as director of program services faced the considerable challenge of creating a wide range of new responses to resident needs. "Places like Pineland had been trampling over patient rights," she said some years later. "Now we were doing something about it, thanks to that decree."

Direct care workers could also bring enthusiasm to the cause. Elaine Gallant was a psychiatric aide who joined the staff at Pineland—where her father and four

Deinstitutionalization is a recent "buzz word" seemingly the in-trend and considered to be spurred on by individuals motivated by humanistic considerations. The issue of deinstitutionalization becomes clouded for many of us because not everyone uses this word to mean the same thing. The extremists are using this term as a movement to close down any and all institutions. Most people in the field, however, think of reconstructing institutions into living units which reflect the standards of good taste, sanitation, safety, privacy, and dignity when they use the term deinstitutionalization. Personally, I choose the latter definition.

—Victor Gartner, assistant to the superintendent, in the winter 1982 Observer

brothers also worked—right after graduating from high school in 1973. At that point, some patients still wore institutional nylon clothing, and conditions were often rough, she remembered in the year 2000. But Pineland improved while Gallant was on a break from 1975 to 1978. The place had "changed a whole lot," she found on her return. "It was a wonderful place and it kept on changing, and it wasn't just the consent decree. That helped, but mostly it was the people."

Superintendent Zitnay told a reporter from *The Maine Paper* much the same thing in 1980:

> *The staff has been fantastic and it all boils down to a matter of pride. We don't have bed sores at Pineland because we take the effort to make certain everyone, even the most severely retarded, has a program and isn't allowed to stay in a bed all day. We don't put catheters on any of our patients. We don't do any intravenous feedings, and the use of medication has dropped drastically. My colleagues who operate institutions in other states are astounded when I tell them that. The reason is a simple one— the staff here takes the extra time to get people out of bed, to help them eat, to change them.*

But would such effort be enough for the court? Tension was high in late spring 1980. With the court's two-year deadline fast approaching, Pineland officials insisted that they were doing all they could; the court master insisted that this was not enough. Something had to give, and it did.

A New Master

In July 1980, U.S. District Court Judge Edward T. Gignoux extended the consent decree for two more years, thus easing the threat of a takeover. In November he appointed a new court master. Gone was David D. Gregory, the man the *Maine Times* described as "a fierce enforcer" of the decree. Moving into position was Lincoln Clark, a professor emeritus from the Graduate School of Business Administration at New York University and an experienced mediator. He approached the job as a gentle encourager. "He was Gignoux's bridge partner," said Jeff Lee, a lawyer looking back from the year 2000 to the 1980s when he was a resident advocate. "Everybody knew his job was to try and settle this thing."

Clark quickly and openly expressed his hope that Pineland would be in full compliance with the decree by July 1981, a year earlier than the new deadline. He

MY SPECIAL BOY
Two big blue eyes, one tiny nose
A crop of light brown hair
A dimpled chin, two cheeks of rose
A smile that knows we care.
Two loving arms, tho' not too strong
A torso ever so slight
Two crippled legs, with feet so wrong
A heart that loves with all its might.
Put them together, one tiny boy
Striving beyond his means
'Til one fine day, his very first step
A fulfillment of all our dreams.
This sounds so natural, but actually not
It's harder than it may seem
For the little boy I'm talking about
has birthdays of thirteen.
For he's retarded . . . it matters not
We love him with all our heart
Always have . . . and always will
until death us do part.
      Wayne's Mother
        —Pineland Observer, *October, November, December 1977*

had his own optimistic views of Pineland's role, views he shared through the *Observer*:

> *Pineland seems to be regarded less and less as an institution for the long term care of the retarded and more and more as an institute for specialized services to prospective parents, new parents, parents of residents, and last but not least, the residents. For example, Pineland has pioneered in genetic research and in counseling prospective parents—and every discovery begets a demand for deeper research. Pineland's counseling of new parents of retarded children is a wonderful supportive service that is bound to increase. Parents when visiting Pineland are thrilled when they see how their children have learned to do something new or better. Many parents have testified that their children seem happier as a result of recent innovations by the Pineland staff. With rapid growth in the number of community homes, much training of personnel is needed and is being increasingly provided by Pineland staff both in the community and at Pineland. . . .*
>
> *For example, there are persons in other state institutions who, if brought to Pineland, could benefit by Pineland's expertise with rehabilitative services, and prospective nurses and social workers might be enrolled in educational programs on the Pineland campus and housed in some of Pineland's buildings.*
>
> *Do the predicted new emphases mean that the Pineland population will continue to decline? Certainly not. If the introduction of new programs and services is synchronized with the transfers of some Pineland residents [with unusual] medical and psychological problems that can be handled better at Pineland than in the community, there could be several new categories of residents in addition to the mentally retarded. . . .*

Clark's prediction of early compliance proved more accurate than his vision for Pineland's future. On September 18, 1981, Gignoux freed Pineland from the jurisdiction of his court.

A Moment of Triumph

"You should be proud of what you've accomplished," the judge told thirty employees of the center and the state Bureau of Mental Retardation he had asked to stand. "I'm sure you'll continue your very good work."

Feelings were cordial and supportive in the courtroom. Neville Woodruff, the plaintiff's attorney who had filed the original suit, was among those voicing positive thoughts. In 1976 he had spoken of "acute boredom, physical deterioration,

I can tell you one funny thing that happened at Pineland when I was there. At least it seems funny now, but I was bonkers then. [A young staff member had signed a Pineland bus out for Sebago Lake State Park, then taken his six charges instead to an X-rated drive-in movie.] He thought it would be therapeutic. I kept waiting for the phone to ring and for people who had seen that bus with the Pineland name on it to complain. But I guess they didn't want to admit that they were at the drive-in. [The staff member was later suspended, then reinstated and reduced in rank.] I was mighty, mighty unhappy.
—*Kevin Concannon, Maine commissioner of Human Services, looking back in January 2001*

social regression, physical debilitation, severe depression, and low morale" among residents. But the years of effort had altered things greatly. "I am fully satisfied that none of those conditions now exists at Pineland," he told the court as it prepared to relinquish control.

Parents of Pineland residents were also present in the court, and one of them, Pennie Whitney of Kittery Point, read a poem about the "friends, not strangers" who had cared for her son at Pineland. "I don't believe Henry Wadsworth Longfellow could have done better," responded Gignoux.

The release from supervision applied only to Pineland itself, not to the state's care of Pineland clients living outside the center. Even so, it was a remarkable accomplishment of national scope, for this was the first time that a federal court had removed itself from such a case. "Over the past decade federal courts have issued a score or more decrees to improve conditions in state institutions for the mentally retarded," said Clark. "Maine is the first state in the nation to achieve compliance with such a decree."

"It was a big change," said Joseph M. Ferri, superintendent in the mid 1980s. Before the class action suit, he remembered in the year 2000, he and other staff members would visit other institutions—in Connecticut, for example—and "they all seemed years ahead of us." Then, after the suit, "it seemed we had advanced ten years over them."

The transformation was partly philosophical, partly procedural, partly physical. "Just taking out the pens made a big difference," according to Ferri. He was referring to the areas surrounded by chain link fences that confined residents outside buildings such as Kupelian Hall on warm days.

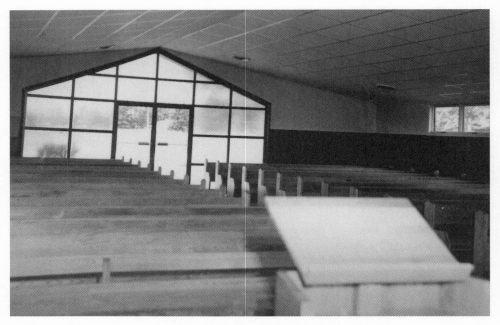

Inside the chapel (courtesy of the New Gloucester Historical Society)

The national Joint Commission on Accreditation of Hospitals added its stamp of approval to the developing institution by fully accrediting Pineland in September 1982.

Fourteen months later in November 1983, the court ended its supervision of community care outside Pineland. That settlement had remained in doubt until late October, when the federal government agreed to a waiver allowing Maine the use of $10 million in Medicaid funds to create 400 new "community beds" so clients could live outside Pineland. Of these, 180 were for use by people still waiting to leave the campus. Again Lincoln Clark was pleased. Compliance might not mean that all 1,000 people covered by the suit were yet receiving every single service mentioned in the decree, he told Gignoux in a letter signed also by the attorneys for plaintiffs and defendants, but:

> It means that "all systems are go," and that nothing in the state's system of care and services impedes full realization of decreed rights to each plaintiff. . . .
>
> Maine now has an excellent system of care for its mentally retarded citizens and I am confident that it will become even better in the years ahead.

Pineland had achieved a high point in its long, sometimes troublesome history. Free at last of direct court control, praised from all sides, it must have been the momentary envy of health care advocates and administrators all over the country. But pinnacles are dangerous, impermanent places for people and institutions to stand, and time would not be still for Pineland. The center could enjoy its moment of satisfaction, but with its population down and its expenses up, it was already on course toward a difficult end.

The Plant

The competing forces of growth and decline were apparent in the condition of Pineland's physical plant. Much was positive; even the center's fleet of sixty vehicles had been upgraded. "As a result of the class action suit, three additional vehicles will be purchased within the next year," said the *Observer* in January 1978. "The first will be a standard school bus, the second will be a 12- or 15-passenger van exclusively for the transportation of wheelchair clients, and the third a standard 12-passenger van." Money would be used for the purchase; apparently nobody suggested that collecting more trading stamps would satisfy the court.

Superintendent Zitnay summarized major plant improvements under way in the fall 1980 edition of the *Observer*:

> *I am happy to report that renovations and improvements in the physical plant at Pineland Center continue to be accomplished. Recently, two, six bed apartments were opened in the Federation Village which were converted by the Maintenance Department at Pineland. Perhaps you have seen the roofing repairs to the Conference Center, to Hedin, Vosburgh Hall,*

Pineland Parents & Friends used the occasion of its first fall meeting on October 12, 1986 to honor Senator Walter Hichens upon his retirement from the State Legislature. Senator Hichens has long been a good and active friend of P.P.F.A., and has repeatedly shown his concern for the welfare of the retarded citizens of his district and of the whole state of Maine. For several years, while Pineland was undergoing many changes in policy and direction, Senator Hichens served as Chairman of the Legislature's Health and Institute Committee, and in the position he was called upon by many Pineland parents and staff to try to find solutions and solve problems. He was always willing to listen, and went out of his way to keep interested parties advised of what was going on.

—Pineland Observer, *November 1986*

In 1985, a fully equipped woodworking shop was built as part of the Behavior Stabilization Unit. The concept was to teach appropriate use of tools, and to provide useful vocation skills to some BSU residents.

In June of 1987, a 19 year old was admitted to the BSU. He had a history of running away and aggression. He also had a desire to do woodworking and a dream of doing something important. In September, a group of residents voiced their concern for two ducks who had taken up residence on Witham Pond. The residents were worried about the ducks getting cold. They wanted the ducks to have a house for the coming winter.

The matter was referred to the BSU and in October these events came together. The BSU would build a duckhouse. One very excited resident made and remade plans. He envisioned a floating duckhouse on a rope and pulley retrieval system. He envisioned a house fully insulated with a hinged roof to facilitate cleaning. Plans were made. Supplies were ordered from the carpentry shop. The floats and pulley system disappeared in the Yankee spirit of simplicity. Staff and resident went to work laminating layers of plywood and foam insulation.

Out by Witham Pond now stands a simple but proud, fully insulated shingle roofed duckhouse. Now a young man feels a little more confident, a bit more grown up, and a whole lot more important.

—Pineland Observer, *winter 1988*

and Cumberland Hall. The most exciting renovation recently completed was the upstairs activity center in the Commons Building. This renovation made possible the closing of New Gloucester Hall and provides for a most attractive and conducive environment for the residents in the Day Activity Center. Soon, a cafeteria will be opened in the Commons Building so that residents participating in the Day Activity Center will be able to have lunch there. This will provide the residents with a good learning experience. Currently underway is the development of the lower floor of the Commons Building which will house a pre-vocational training center as well as offices for some of the professional staff. An elevator is in the process of being built to connect the two floors and to provide access for all clients. These ongoing renovations are part of the continuing commitment to constantly review and improve services to clients at Pineland.

With the completion of its renovation in 1981, the Commons Building was rededicated and renamed as the Governor James B. Longley Center.

Pineland's population at the time of Zitnay's report was 330 residents, but the plant received more use than the number suggested, because the center had served 2,000 people on an outpatient basis the previous year, providing such things as dental care, X-rays, genetic counseling, lab work, and consultations.

The refurbished physical plant impressed a writer for *The Maine Paper* in July 1980:

> *The traditional symbols of mental institutions have been eliminated. The drab wards with their rows of cots and barred windows have been replaced by apartments which one would expect to find in a good motel or at an exclusive girls' school. Six well-supervised retarded adults share an apartment which is carpeted and decorated to individual tastes. Each contains a sitting area with neat and attractive furniture, including television and stereo equipment. Some of the apartments have kitchen and dining areas and the residents participate in the preparation of their meals.*

Building changes continued throughout the decade as new programs began and old ones ended. In fact the library's location switched so often that its movement became a bit of a joke. A testimony written for one-time librarian Rose P. Ricker at her 1983 retirement said in part:

> *Then a strange phenomenon began to occur. Her stable library program suddenly became a moving library, a sort of book mobile without wheels. During a course of several years, books spent more time in moving*

This year is the 10th anniversary of the Consent Decree, and also Pineland Center's 80th birthday. It is a time to assess the progress made, the difficulties overcome, and the challenges to be met in the coming months and years.

The current plan to reorganize Pineland into clusters is an example of meeting one of those major challenges. It reflects the identified needs of residents to have consistency and continuity in their lives, as we all do, in order to achieve their greatest potential. The development of six interdisciplinary teams will enable a consistent and cohesive group of staff members to work with a consistent group of residents over time. Program and residential staff will work together to ensure appropriate services for the entire waking day, so that each resident can progress along the continuum to less restrictive care and greater independence.

—*Superintendent Spencer Moore in the* Pineland Observer, *winter 1988*

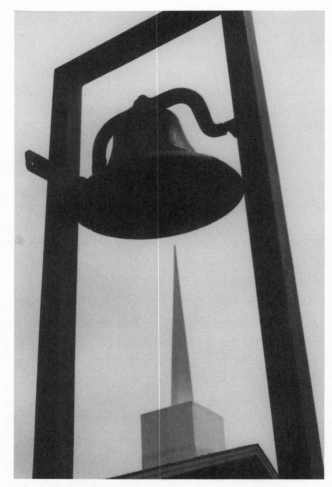

Chapel bell and steeple (courtesy of Elaine Gallant)

cartons than on shelves. Staff were generally confused as to which build-
ing to go to for library help. During this period of time the library was
located (not necessarily in chronological order):

*   - In the downstairs part of Berman School*
*   - Where the Adult Learning Center program now is in the Longley*
*   Center*
*   - Where the Personnel Department now is in Hedin*
*   - Where the Superintendent's complex now is in Hedin*
*   - Where the Housekeeping complex now is in Hedin basement—and*
*   - A long time ago, where the library currently is in Staff development*

Plant changes could have great significance for residents and their programs. The opening of the therapeutic pool attached to the Soucy gym was an example. Darla Chafin, a longtime member and occasional president of Pineland Parents and Friends, remembered its initial impact several years after Pineland closed. "That warm water did wonders," she said. "It relaxed people, loosened them. One 45-year-old man who had never spoken in his life stood there in that water and said, 'I want to get out now.'"

But despite all this, elsewhere on the campus were signs of closure, indications of deterioration. New Gloucester Hall was already empty in 1983 when Superintendent Zitnay announced that "eventually Vosburgh Hall will be closed as a residential building, since it is the oldest building still in use that has not been renovated and Pownal Hall will be closed as a program site since with fewer clients we can do a better job of programming with fewer physical plants to maintain."

Zitnay thought that New Gloucester Hall should be preserved as a museum, complete with the bars on its windows, and told a visiting reporter:

> *We think it is important for people to see the way things were when this was known as an insane asylum or a school for the feeble-minded. Once there were rows of cots lining both sides of this room and people came here and just lay in them. This building once housed 90 residents. I think it's important to preserve New Gloucester Hall as a reminder of the dark days. It will keep us from forgetting and keep us moving forward.*

But that was not to happen. Although New Gloucester Hall did become a storage site for court documents, it continued to decay along with other parts of the campus. In 1986, Governor Joseph E. Brennan appointed a task force to consider new uses for empty buildings, and the Maine State Police canine training program moved onto the campus in 1987. But such new arrivals never fully compensated for the continuing departure of residents.

Sunday, August 14, 1983

Started to clean out the fridge—it proved to be one of the strangest experiences I have had at P. C. I'll bet no lab on the east coast has this many cultures growing—slimy flat green tomatoes, a large green fuzzy sandwich, breads of several types that could be used for hockey pucks, and several items that I couldn't identify. Also a jar of water (?) that had white cloudy stuff in the bottom and black mold floating on top. One very foul smelling carton of milk. I gave up at this point.

—*Shift supervisor's log*

Peter W. Bowman, M.D., superintendent of Pineland Hospital and Training Center from 1953–1971, was honored at the presentation of a portrait for display in the Administration Building. The portrait was commissioned in 1986 by a group of organizations and individuals to honor Dr. Bowman for his many achievements at Pineland Center and for his leadership in his professional field.

—Pineland Observer, *1987*

A Developing System

As Pineland's useful physical plant became smaller, so did its role in the state's system of care for people with retardation. Outside the grounds and around the state, many community residences—nursing homes, boardinghouses, family care homes, group homes, supervised apartment programs, and intermediate care facilities—were appearing. Usually operating with the assistance of federal and state money and supervision, the new facilities offered beds to Pineland clients and others and often gave them a chance to live closer to friends and family.

One new nonresidential program, the Southern Maine Resource Center, had taken offices in the old administration building on the Pineland campus in 1978. Its purpose was providing services to developmentally disabled people living in the community. Another new program moved away from its birthplace at Pineland to nearby Freeport.

Residents in Pineland's Sheltered Workshop Program, which provided services to local businesses, had for several years been located in the Bliss Workshop and the Work Activities Center. The program's operation was spawned partly by court decisions that residents must be paid fair wages for work performed and partly by the fact that Pineland lacked funds to make such payment. Hooking up with outside industry was a reasonable answer, and residents in the program now made partitions for Ellis Paperboard Products of Portland and "Lunch Snack" packages for Circus Time Potato Chips. They packed soap and toothbrushes for Tom's of Maine and did mailings for the W. S. Libby Company of Lewiston. They also earned substantial amounts of money—$75,000 in one year, said Kevin Concannon, director of the Bureau of Mental Retardation.

In 1979 the Sheltered Workshop moved to the old Freeport Towne Square building, purchased by the state from a furniture company. Twelve residents of Pineland would live in the new location, Concannon said as he announced the move, and fifty more would be bused in daily to work on various contracted projects.

Sixteen months after the move, Charles E. Fairweather, the workshop's procurement specialist, proclaimed it a success in the *Observer*. Staff members had used some ingenuity to counter the effects of a national economic slump, and the workshop was measuring its operations in the millions. Employees had assembled 4 million components for Ellis, for example, and performed 1.25 million operations on trick-or-treat bags for the Nissen Baking Company.

In November 1985, the program expanded and became the Martti A. Wuori Workshop, dedicated to the memory of the resident whose name had been given symbolically to the class action suit of the 1970s. In 1989 the workshop celebrated its tenth anniversary and saw some of its employees providing housekeeping services for a local motel.

Meanwhile, Back on the Campus

Despite the activity elsewhere, things were still humming at the center. Having six programmed hours for every resident every day meant lots of planning, lots of training and therapy, lots of classes, lots of movement.

Beginning in the spring of 1980, a concept called "Interfacing" helped smooth the movement of residents and staff around the campus. As explained in 1984 by Marion Cromwell, a coordinator of volunteer services, the concept led program staff, teachers, teacher aides, therapists, and therapy aides to begin their workday by reporting first to residential units and assisting staff there in getting residents ready to attend daily programming. In turn, residential staff accompanied residents to the program sites and remained with them through the program hours. The concept "has proven very beneficial," said Cromwell. "It has ensured that each resident's individual treatment plan is carried out with continuity throughout the day. At the same time, it has improved communications among a variety of staff—and an appreciation for one another's job."

Virtually all program areas changed significantly during the decade, and the Berman School was no exception. From its opening in 1958, it provided classes in conventional subjects to Pineland's school-age population and to some day students from outside. Although its students had special needs, it operated and looked

> Pineland was good for the kids in a lot of ways. For one thing, nobody laughed at them there. I never saw anybody laugh at anybody. I never saw anybody made fun of.
> —*Nancy Wilcox, one-time Pineland employee, remembering back from the year 2000*

like a typical American public school building. But as Pineland's population changed, the residents most suited to such training moved into community programs. Those who remained had more severe conditions, often multiple handicaps requiring a different space and a different staff response. In the fall of 1983, the Berman School closed and its programs moved across Morse Road from the central campus to Perry Hayden Hall. There the staff included teachers, physical and occupational therapists and aides, a mental retardation trainer, a recreation aide, mental health workers, three foster grandmothers, and a principal. Suzanne Lausier was the principal in 1984; reflecting back on the change, she said in the *Observer*:

> *We appreciate the process that has taken our former students back to their rightful place, living and working in our communities. We know that much has been done to build the resources needed to keep students (no matter what their needs) in their community schools, thus ensuring that they grow up among family and friends. This is our hope for the students of the New Perry Hayden School that the services and supports that they and their families need are a natural part of this historic process.*

Pineland offered new classes for staff members as well as residents in the 1980s. Some were training programs designed to advance job skills. Others were more general in nature. Beginning in 1980, for example, the University of Maine offered a three-year program leading to an associate of science degree.

Moments of Pleasure

Not all the center's staff and resident hours were devoted to serious pursuits such as training and finding new community homes. In the 1980s, as in some earlier years, significant energy went into entertainment and recreation around the calendar. Late in the decade, when the *Observer* had shrunk to a four-page bimonthly filled largely with positive news of interest to Pineland family and

---

Ferri presented a plaque, which will hang in the foyer of the Administration Building at Pineland, as a token of gratitude to the Founders [of Camp Tall Pines]. The plaque carries an inscription taken from the works of Henry David Thoreau: "To affect the quality of the day, that is the highest of the arts." It was unanimously agreed that the Camp Tall Pines Foundation has "affected the quality of the day" for many, many developmentally disabled citizens of Maine.

—Pineland Observer *report of an award ceremony at Tall Pines in October 1983*

Keep the resident behind a locked door long enough and you can then unlock the door and they won't know what to do . . . At least that has seemed to be the case in our unit. When we all first came to Cumberland Hall as part of "the change," we were different aides and different residents getting used to one another. We were also comprised of three wards with unlocked, open doors, but you would never have known it. Most residents would come to the open door and stop automatically—as though it were still locked. Or one of us aides would unconsciously call out, "Come back here!" Talk about being conditioned! It would be interesting to ponder who was more conditioned—aides or residents.

But gradually we all relaxed and learned freedom, even if it only involved one floor of one building. One girl would discover she could actually walk through that door and go visiting in another ward, or just walk back and forth in a hall and look into different rooms or out of different windows. As the days passed, the boys and girls would timidly venture into another ward, and we aides lost the compulsion to say, "Get back to your ward."

—Sharon Malthy, reporter, Cumberland Hall I, in the Pineland Observer, *January, February 1974*

friends, many issues had half or more of their space devoted to photographs and stories of recreational events.

Fall saw full-costume Halloween parties and other celebrations such as the Very Special Arts Festival of 1988. Parents, friends, and past employees joined residents and staff at that event to mark Pineland's eightieth birthday with painting, sculpting, silk-screening, and music-making activities.

The winter season began with rounds of holiday parties and continued, weather permitting, with festivals including outdoor sports and snow sculpture competitions. Valentine's Day parties featured the naming of two residents as King and Queen of Hearts, and the Special Olympics had residents competing in swimming, bowling, basketball, and outdoor sports.

The warming months were celebrated with spring festivals. In 1990, paddleboats carried residents and friends across Witham Pond, and a horse-drawn wagon took them around the grounds. Just outside Soucy gym, clients flew kites, created spatter paintings, and made butter, bubbles, and ice cream. The spring celebrations of the early 1980s included more Very Special Arts Festivals, using funds provided by the National Committee on Arts for the Handicapped to the Maine State Commission on the Arts and the Humanities, and culminated with such year-round art activities as artist-in-residency programs, workshops, and training conferences.

Summer brought another round of Special Olympics and visits to Tall Pines. But the events remembered best by many Pineland workers, residents, and friends were the Independence Day celebrations. "I remember them since I was a kid," said Elaine Gallant in 2000. "They were great." They had long been important, and they remained so through the 1980s, with bands and fire companies and entertainers from local communities. The *Observer* enthused over the 1989 event:

> Pineland's 4th of July Celebration belonged to the best in everyone, the child.
>
> Dozens of individual efforts came together to create a magical bubble where personal concerns could be suspended. . . .
>
> From the opening ceremonies at the bandstand to the last notes of the Summit Spring Band the day lived up to the anticipation of it. The Indian Tribal Dance performed by the Pineland Aerobics Group delighted the crowd as much as the participants. The Heart of Gold Vaudeville Show held people riveted until it was time for the legendary chicken barbeque. The kitchen staff served a record number of delicious meals to an appreciative throng.
>
> The parade exceeded expectations. Seventeen residential units entered floats in the parade. They were imaginative and beautifully constructed.

Volunteer Services

Volunteers were important to the special events at Pineland. But volunteers were also important every day throughout the institution. Some made substantial contributions for years. One of these was Mrs. Grace Self, who had first worked at the school with her late husband, Frank, in the early 1950s. Thirty years later she was honored for her contributions to many of the major volunteer projects of three decades—providing Christmas gifts; collecting stamps to use in buying a bus; raising funds for the chapel, gym, and swimming pool; and leading the Frank D. Self Foundation, which had supported numerous research and other projects at the center.

A new volunteer effort began in 1983, according to the *Observer*, when a volunteer from the local Retired Senior Volunteer Program "came to Pineland looking for something worthwhile to do in his retirement and recognized the hidden potential within his assigned group of residents." The volunteer was William Norton, and his assigned group was elderly Pineland residents. They soon formed their own chapter of RSVP, and their project was making Christmas angels out of

NEW GLOUCESTER—It really is a perfect friendship in an odd sort of way.

Fred will accept almost nothing and Eddy-Brophy Campbell has little to give but a friendship sealed in a letter each month.

They've never met. They've never spoken. It's likely they never will. Fred will never leave the Pineland Center for the Mentally Retarded here. Campbell is serving a 55-year sentence in prison. . . .

For a year, Campbell has been Fred's "correspondent," a relationship that demands much more than the letters he mails once a month.

A correspondent is a friend, someone who steps in to help retarded persons who have no active relatives or guardians. Although it's neither a legal nor a financial commitment, it is an emotional one. Most correspondents see their friend regularly, perhaps take him or her out to dinner or shopping, get to know the staff that works with him, and try to safeguard his interests when plans are made for treatment or services.

But Fred and Campbell's friendship is a "very unusual one." Campbell can't do all those things and Fred wouldn't allow them, even if he could.

Fred lives an inner life at which others can only guess. Originally from Androscoggin County, he will soon be 75 and he's spent 65 of those years at Pineland.

—*Article by Roberta Scruggs, Sunday staff writer,*
Maine Sunday Telegram, *February 17, 1985*

heavy paper. The RSVP members did the initial work stamping and cutting angel faces for assembly by the Freeport Towne Square Sheltered Workshop. Hannaford Brothers stepped in at that point and sold the angels through the popular "Be an Angel–Buy an Angel" project. By December 1985, about 45,000 angels had found their way into Maine homes. That year Hannaford presented the center a check for $15,000, which meant profits of $5,000 that could be used for building a theater. The next year, 50,000 angels produced a check for $25,000 and a profit of $8,000.

Among the best-publicized volunteer efforts for Pineland was the annual relay, run by the Maine Rowdy Running Team. Its members solicited pledges to benefit Pineland, then ran the 400 miles from Fort Kent to Kittery in 20-mile segments. These were serious running enthusiasts—their number at one point included Olympian Joan Benoit—and they were successful. By 1985 they had raised a total of $40,000 for the center. They also surprised some observers along the way. The

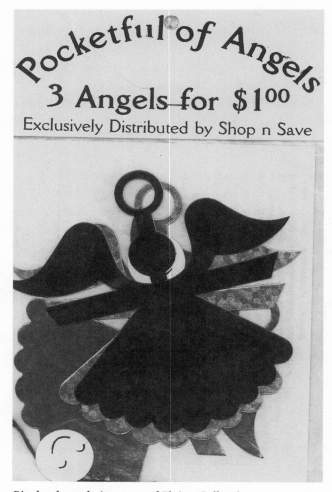

Pineland angels (courtesy of Elaine Gallant)

first runner and the last had send-off and welcoming committees, but others had no such support, said the *Observer*.

> *After the first few miles, it becomes a lone runner followed by a trail car. Occasionally a car will draw alongside the runner and someone will yell out, "Where are you running to"? Over his shoulder, as he keeps his stride, the response is "Kittery." This reply draws mixed reactions—especially if it is three in the morning—somewhere near Mars Hill.*

Some of Pineland's most committed volunteers were members of the center's staff, working on their own time. Many of them did it, by all accounts, often to the

I remember one girl who went to all the services. She went to the rabbi's service on Friday and to mass on Saturday. Sunday she went to protestant services. Somebody asked her about that once and she explained why she did it. "When I go to heaven I don't know what door is going to be open, and I want to be ready."

—Nancy Wilcox, one-time Pineland employee, remembering back from the year 2000

direct benefit of residents. Rose Ricker was one of them; she and her husband sometimes opened their Buckfield farm to camping trips by residents, including six men from Valley View Farm, a building on Morse Road near the Pineland campus. The six had all been institutionalized for long periods and had behavioral maladjustments, said Ricker in an article she wrote for the *Observer* (without identifying the farm or the effort as hers), and their first two trips were a great success:

It all sounds so simple—and so desirable, if only one could see how these residents respond to a relaxed, lots-of-space, non-pressured environment, even if it means quite primitive living.

One forty-plus resident, who's lived at Pineland for over 20 years, and who strenuously resists any change in his routine, now goes quite willingly when he's told he's "going camping."

But the red tape and paperwork involved is ridiculous! Something that is so normal and healthy for residents and staff alike should have top priority, but frequently is fraught with road blocks. So be it—we keep talking about normalization and community interaction, but we don't always work to make this possible. My hat's off to the Valley View staff, who have persisted in trying to enrich the lives of their residents.

Wayne P. Haskell shared Ricker's interest in helping residents beyond the campus limits. As an aide at the Children's Psychiatric Hospital in the 1960s, he became very attached to one patient, a fourteen-year-old boy. In time the boy became Haskell's foster son and lived with him for a year, supported only by the state's meager contribution of seventy-nine dollars a month. Their relationship continued for decades; in the year 2001, with the former patient now a forty-two year old, they remained in close touch.

> The [consent] decree . . . guaranteed residents a right to individualized treatment in the most normal, least restrictive setting possible. By state policy, that guarantee extends to all Maine's mentally retarded citizens.
>
> But Maine is never going to make good on that promise unless the money poured into the state's aged institution in Pownal is liberated for community services, say a growing number of people familiar with the issue.
>
> —Maine Times, *December 15, 1989*

Special Grandparents

A group of "almost volunteers" were Pineland's Foster Grandparents. Their presence began at the center in 1972, when people who were sixty years old and within certain income limits agreed to work four hours a day, five days a week in return for a small stipend. Each was to spend two hours a day with each of two children, and they soon were giving more and receiving more than the size of their stipend suggested. Said the *Observer* in 1978:

> *Very few grandparents quit. To date, Pineland's twenty Foster Grandparents have contributed 63,000 hours of service. Many have been with the same child for the past six years. This is very important since there has been considerable staff turnover in the past. For some residents, the foster grandparent has been the most constant familiar face for as long as they can remember.*

Through the 1980s, the program developed and expanded. Betty Wurtz, wife of former Pineland superintendent Conrad Wurtz, was a regional coordinator in Maine's version of the national program. In 1987, when three Foster Grandparents were serving the center, she wrote for the *Observer*:

> *Love, friendship, attention and care! Talking, touching, sharing and helping! Giving an example of living skills to kids who need them. Receiving the intangible rewards of helping others. That's what the Foster Grandparent Program is about.*
>
> *Maine's approximately 72 Foster Grandparents are located in over 20 sites around the state. For four hours a day, five days a week, they provide love, attention and help for over 170 children and young adults with special educational and social needs. They read stories to the youngsters, assist with meals, play games with them, provide tutoring services, and generally help the kids with a wide variety of other projects. Even more importantly,*

the program provides an opportunity for young people to experience first-hand learning of values and a chance for both the younger and older generations to form lasting and meaningful relationships.

New Troubles

But all the volunteer efforts and all the love and all the goodwill created by settlement of the Martti Wuori case could not protect Pineland from a new round of problems. They hit the news in mid-decade with the publication of articles written by editor and reporter Lance Tapley for "Coping," a newsletter published by the Maine Association of Handicapped Persons.

Tapley's articles grew out of weeks spent reviewing allegations of staff abuse at Pineland since 1982. Institutional reforms required by the consent decree had established new procedures for tracking responses to reports of abuse. From early 1982 until the time of his article, there had been 137 such reports, some indicating such serious matters as a death that might have involved negligence, an employee forcefully dunking a resident's head in the pool, a worker and a resident found naked in a locked closet, and physical assault. The complaints had been handled largely in-house, Tapley charged, when in fact they should have been reported to the attorney general's office.

Also, said "Coping," Pineland's new Behavior Stabilization Unit had a "prison-like atmosphere" and was "beset with problems."

The Consumer Advisory Board, set up to monitor Pineland, was ineffectual, according to an unnamed state official who claimed, said "Coping," that the board could only write letters. "There's no recourse," the official said. "It's like having a

There are very few children at the Pineland Center now, said John Hoffman, a social research scientist at the center since 1962.

The children there, he explained, "tend to be older children and they tend to be very, very severely physically handicapped."

In an institution, he continued, "there isn't the emotional . . . support that children should get. The feeling is that the child isn't going to develop . . . and to my mind it's very harmful."

A mentally retarded child born in the state of Maine runs among the least risks of being institutionalized of children anywhere in the nation, agreed Ned Graham, case work supervisor for the Bureau of Mental Retardation.

—Kennebec Journal, *June 2, 1986*

wiffle baseball bat." Board chair Mickey Boutilier refuted that opinion; others protested the entire "Coping" exposé.

The articles were "the kind of journalism you find at the supermarket checkout counter," said Mental Health commissioner Concannon.

"The people who drafted this article have no idea the devastation this has caused," charged Charles L. Wyman. A retired naval officer and the father of a Pineland resident, Wyman had played an important role at Pineland as Governor James B. Longley's special assistant and in various volunteer capacities since then. Tapley should have taken the time to visit a Human Rights Committee meeting, Wyman said. "It gives you a great deal of assurance there are no allegations swept under the rug."

But the charges did not fade away. The attorney general's office began an investigation, and the *Maine Times* renewed its interest in Pineland. It reported two deaths in October that raised the possibility of neglect, one in which a resident swallowed a safety pin, which punctured his lung, and another in which a resident choked on peanut butter while unattended.

Later that fall, Attorney General James Tierney concluded that the system of reporting abuse was "working well" overall, but the *Maine Times* was having none of that. "How could the system have been working well when the law was not being followed, not even by Tierney's own office?" the paper asked in a December article under the headline "COPING IS VINDICATED."

A piece of good news hit the papers in January 1986, when Pineland was accredited for another three years by the Joint Commission on Accreditation of Hospitals. But another death occurred in February when a resident wandered into the woods and succumbed. His body was not found for two days, and an investigation concluded that "major systems failures" occurred in the search for him. The panel urged the discipline of several employees. The group did not include Superintendent Ferri, but in April Ferri decided it was time for him to step down and continue his service to the school in other capacities.

November 18, 1985

J_ T_ became very upset when asked to go in living room, sitting technique used, security officer called, J_ was put in T.O. [time out] chair, he broke his watch, glasses and a lamp, he also bit R_M_ on index finger, left hand, scratched R_s left leg, also. J_ will have a black eye - received the injury during the time he was being restrained. Took 2 unit staff plus both S. officers to restrain him.

—*Shift supervisor's log*

1. Maine has the 8th lowest placement rate per 100,000 population with a rate of 24.58 [placed in state institutions] compared to a national average of 42.0,
2. Maine has the 4th lowest incidence of placement of persons with mild or moderate retardation. These two categories make up only 8.7% of the population in Maine's state operated facilities,
3. In 1987 Maine had the 2nd highest rate of returning people to the community who had been readmitted to a state operated facility, and
4. Maine has the 9th highest daily costs per resident, $188.36 per day compared to a national average of $149.36.

—Findings in a University of Minnesota study of state institutions and people with retardation, for the year ending June 30, 1987

"I'm the sort of person who thinks that anything happens on your watch you're responsible for," Ferri said a decade and a half after the event. "This happened on my watch."

In 1987 came the news that a jury had found an eighty-two-year-old Yarmouth physician, who was on duty at the center in 1983, negligent for his response to a heart attack that had taken the life of a Pineland employee.

As this series of reports was appearing, the value of Pineland's Behavioral Stabilization Unit (BSU) was being publicly debated. The fifteen-bed BSU had opened in the winter of 1984 to house mentally retarded people with significant behavioral problems. The state needed the unit, said Commissioner Concannon, because community facilities could not handle violent outbursts. "Mentally retarded people were showing up in jails and the jails couldn't treat them." So the BSU took on the job using controversial behavioral modification techniques combined with what staffers said was tight control and full record keeping. Employees at the unit rewarded patients for good behavior by punching cards, allowing them to buy candy, play pinball, or go on outings. Punishments used for bad behavior increased gradually, Ferri told the *Press Herald* in 1986.

For causing minor disruptions, patients had to leave the group and sit quietly for about ten minutes. Those who caused more serious problems spent up to an

The thing I feared the most as a shift supervisor was a lost resident.
—Wayne Haskell, looking back from the year 2000

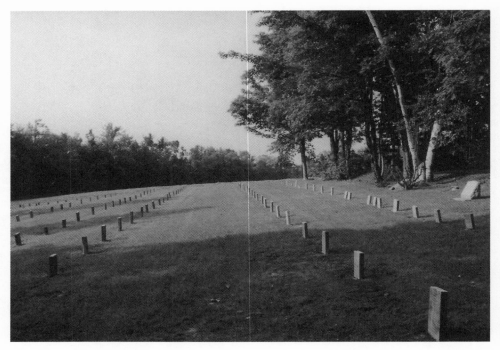

Pineland's cemetery (author photo)

hour alone in a supervised room. Dangerous actions meant being strapped, while under observation, for up to an hour in a restraint chair in a dim cinder-block room with a padded floor. Drugs were used as a last resort.

"The BSU was not meant to be attractive," Ferri told the paper. It was designed for short-term stays that would prepare patients for a return to the community.

But some stays were not so short. This worried Rose Ricker, the former librarian who had become chairwoman of Pineland's Human Rights and Assurance Committee. "The BSU isn't operating the way it was intended to. It is supposed to be crisis intervention. But it has been difficult to find places for some people, and others haven't responded as quickly as possible."

> Being superintendent was an extremely consuming job. It was twenty-four hours a day. . . . But the job had some good aspects. You could effect change and that was good. I enjoyed a lot of it.
>
> —*Joseph M. Ferri, looking back from the year 2000*

> The problem still remains of staff discarding cigarette butts on the ground where clients can get them and ingest them.
> —*Executive Management Committee minutes for January 11, 1989*

Parents and clients weighed in on both sides of the controversy, with some praising the BSU in news reports and letters columns, and some condemning it, most basing their opinions on specific cases.

Continuing press probes were difficult for some Pineland staffers to accept. "They were always making us look bad," Elaine Gallant remembered years later. "But we were doing our best. We didn't use restraint chairs for small things. But clients could be rough. In fact one woman broke my nose."

"The papers could be tough, especially the *Maine Times*," said Ferri. "That was always hitting hard, especially on restraints. It looked terrible, I agree. But nobody could give any other idea what to do about really aggressive people and people who really tried to hurt themselves."

The BSU continued to operate through the rest of the decade. Critical press reports continued, too, and as time passed they became more general. There had been some progress at Pineland, but there were now signs of backsliding, said the *Maine Times* in a 1988 article. The account displayed photos of patients being restrained at Kupelian Hall in 1969 and credited the paper itself with helping to start what improvements had been made. "Come on, *Maine Times*, get with it," said a response from Pineland's Board of Visitors. "Your article is a confused, self-serving mass of truth out-of-control."

But such reactions failed to stop the critical reports.

In January 1989, the Consumer Advisory Board concluded that the state was out of compliance with the consent decree in some respects. On May 27 of that year, the *Press Herald* announced that Pineland might lose $10 million a year in Medicaid funds because it "is not meeting several key standards for patient care." By July the staff had resolved the problems, and funds had again been assured. But new complaints were lodged with the Pineland Consent Decree Panel in October by clients who found services wanting. In December the *Press Herald* carried a headline stating, "Abuse complaints on rise at Pineland." The paper corrected itself the next day after discovering that a reporter had erred by comparing statistics from two different sources. The number of complaints investigated by internal review teams had actually decreased—from seventy-six in 1988 to forty-three in

1989. But the articles together must have reinforced a reader perception that whatever the actual number of complaints, abuse still occurred at Pineland.

"Maine's broken promise to mentally retarded: Is Pineland the stumbling block?" read a headline in the *Maine Times* for December 15 of that year.

Pineland's employees felt the downward slide of outside opinion about their workplace. "It was getting so that if you worked there you loved it," said Wayne Haskell. "If you didn't work there you hated it."

Pineland, of course, had experienced and survived difficult periods before. It might have survived this one, too, had all its human energy and all its financial and physical resources been devoted to securing its future. But they were not. Many were devoted to ensuring the center's continuing decline in size. The administrators with the greatest power over Pineland were increasingly asking whether the whole place should not close.

A Darker Horizon

Pineland's resident population was 278 in March 1987 and 267 in January 1989. The decrease had slowed as financial limitations made finding community beds more difficult, but it had not ended.

To the friends and supporters of Pineland who wished to keep the center open, such numbers must have seemed just as large and dark as the cloud that Pinky Karwowski had seen on the horizon in 1980. When they began seeing plans to use the physical plant in alternative ways, a thick and gloomy sky must have closed in around them.

Maybe the vacant buildings should be used for senior citizen housing, suggested Donnell P. Carroll, a state representative from Gray, as he asked for legislative creation of a commission to study such possibilities in 1985. He had already polled his district about the idea with a questionnaire, and he considered the

> The fire is lit, the water is heating in the "Reorganization Locomotive" boiler, and the steam pressure is building! Effective Monday, April 4th, the throttle is thrown forward and the "QMRP wheels" start spinning! On that date, the "Q"s assume their caseload responsibilities for those units, and the assigned residents who will be transferred to those units, as identified on the Final Draft (dated 2/9/88) of the Reorganization Plan Clusters.
>
> *—From a Pineland staff memo concerning a 1988 reorganization plan*

Sunday, Jan. 19th, 1986

S_M_ was missing for a little while this a.m. She left her unit shortly after nine and was headed for the Leisure Center. She never arrived at the L.C. and was seen by security by the Morse House (this was before she was reported "missing"). They told her to head back towards her unit. She didn't. A preliminary search did not locate her. All units were notified to check their areas. At 11:05 S_ returned to the unit. Search concluded. Too bad all searches weren't this easy.

—Shift supervisor's log

response enthusiastic. "There seems to be a good relationship between the senior citizens and the mentally retarded," he told the *Press Herald.*

The next year a legislative committee began considering a new idea: replacing Pineland with five fifty-bed regional centers to serve the state's mentally handicapped. That idea received support from a number of interested parties, including the chair of the Pineland Board of Visitors, Charles L. Wyman. "I was one of those who had to be convinced, and at this point I am convinced, as is the Board of Visitors," he said as state officials showed a model of how such a center might look. "The parents have come to realize that the buildings of Pineland are really getting quite ancient."

Another proposal being studied by the committee proved decidedly less popular. It would have turned Pineland into a minimum- and medium-security prison. Bob Davis, who lived two miles away, was soon knocking on doors asking neighbors to voice their opposition at a meeting with the state's corrections commissioner. "I just don't like criminals in my back yard," Davis told a reporter.

These plans were put aside in 1987 when Governor John R. McKernan, Jr., asked for a long-range-planning study of the regional center concept. Soon after that the Bureau of Public Lands began assessing public interest in using the lands around the central campus for "low intensity" recreation such as walking and picnicking, and Carroll told the *Portland Evening Express* of some other ideas for the campus itself. The buildings could be used for a regional detention center for people convicted of drunk driving, he said, or for an emergency shelter for homeless or battered wives and children.

Pineland residents live in clusters that are determined by their learning and behavioral needs. This grouping means that individual developmental and therapeutic objectives are supported by staff teams. Each resident benefits from a consistent understanding of their needs and the comfort of staff continuity.

AGING CLUSTER

This cluster for the population which is aging . . . strives to provide a responsive environment to meet the unique and changing health, social, emotional, behavioral and sensory needs presented by this population. . . .

THERAPEUTIC CLUSTER

It is the mission of the Therapeutic Cluster to provide care, treatment and training to residents identified as needing specialized nursing care and therapeutic intervention (i. e., occupational, physical, speech, psychological therapy, etc.). . . .

WORK ACTIVITIES CLUSTER

The mission of this cluster is to serve individuals who function with socialization and work skills well above their developmental levels. . . .

PRACTICAL LIFE CLUSTER

The mission of the Practical Life Cluster is to offer training and services which promote the practical and useful application, adaptation, and integration of developmental/behavioral skills necessary for semi-independent or independent daily living. . . .

FUNDAMENTAL/PRACTICAL LIFE CLUSTER

The mission of this cluster is to serve individuals needing care and treatment in the areas of fundamental and practical life skills. . . .

FUNDAMENTAL LIFE CLUSTER

The mission of the Fundamental Life Cluster is the development and enhancement of basic daily living skills.

—Pineland information sheet for visitors in the late 1980s

A Glance Backward

Charles L. Wyman and many others were intent on discussing Pineland's future as the 1980s came to an end. But another Charles Wyman stepped onto the stage in 1989 to speak of the past. He was Charles O. Wyman, the man who had escaped from the grounds sixty-one years before. Now seventy-nine and living in central Maine, he thought of visiting his old institutional home "for sentimental reasons." He spoke to Governor McKernan's secretary, who in turn spoke to Jeff Lee, who was then assistant superintendent. Lee called Wyman and invited him to the center's Independence Day celebration.

History was written when Wyman appeared and told his stories to a fascinated audience. The trees impressed him most, he told a *Press Herald* reporter. "There weren't any big trees like that before."

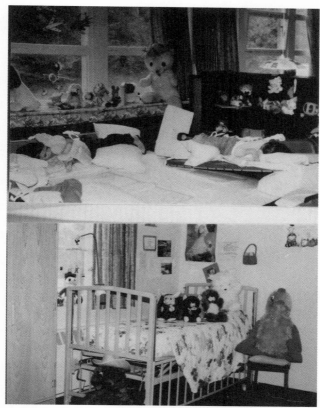

A Pineland pediatrics room (courtesy of the New Gloucester Historical Society)

Wyman also found new approaches to the treatment of residents. "They are awful good to them," he said. "When I was there, they just put them in a corner and left them there."

In fact, Wyman rather liked the place. "I went all around when I was there," he reported. "It's one of the most beautiful places in the state. I got tears in my eyes, I'll tell you."

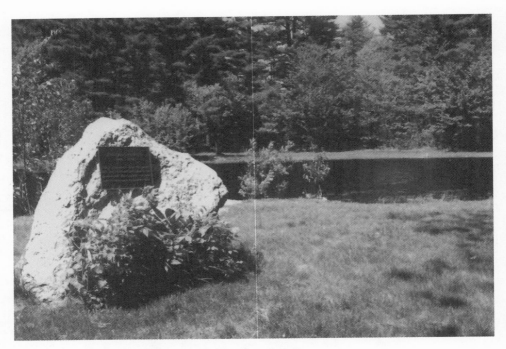

Stone and plaque beside Witham Pond (author photo)

Closure: 7
1990–1996

Change means movement. Movement means friction.
—Saul Alinsky

Feelings about Pineland Center churned and mixed and changed as the 1980s rolled into the 1990s. Government funds were tight to the point of a cost-cutting crisis, and some figures suggested that community placements were a lower-cost alternative to Pineland. Many legislators and administrators believed with increasing intensity that the center should close completely. Others, including many parents, felt an almost urgent need to keep it open. They liked what Pineland was now providing their children, and they distrusted the community option. Still others focused more on the present than the future; they struggled to contain the negative tug of decline as Pineland continued to distance itself in time—and, they said, in spirit—from the consent settlements of 1981 and 1983.

"It's a fallacy to think that the victory is ever won," Neville Woodruff told a 1988 conference celebrating the tenth anniversary of the consent decree. "We could even be losing ground."

Reverend William R. Booth sounded a louder, angrier alarm in the winter 1990 edition of the *Observer*. Booth was chair of Pineland's Board of Visitors, and the *Observer* was quick to say that his views about the policies of the state and Governor John McKernan's administration were his own, not Pineland's. They were also sharply critical:

> *In the wild confusion of our economic troubles, the people of Maine are in danger of losing a sense of proportion. We are being told that we can no longer afford the services of state government at the level to which we have become accustomed. . . .*

195

In the past year . . .Pineland's story, written in Augusta, has been one of reacting without direction to one crisis after another. These crises have included certification problems, budget-cutting proposals, inappropriate admissions, wasting staff resources and the deterioration of services.

Present proposals to cut services in both community centers and Pineland are now reversing progress and leading toward a resumption of outdated, discredited, expensive institution-based programs. . . .

Maine people should call on our governor and legislators to overcome their fears of unpopularity, give up their political game and exercise the authority of their high offices in leading us toward a resolution of this crisis which will do credit to the values of a proud people.

Direct care workers such as Elaine Gallant also detected a backward slide at Pineland. In 1990, Gallant wrote a letter to the *Press Herald* recalling how far the center had progressed since she began to work there in 1973, and expressing concern for the future. "Now, because of state money being low, resulting in layoffs and shortened hours," she said, "I fear the residents will lose their transformed

A RECIPE OF LOVE
1 STAFF
3 RESIDENTS
10 LBS. OF PATIENCE
5 CUPS OF LOVE
6 TSP. OF RELUCTANCE
7 QTS. OF TOLERANCE
6 PTS. OF UNDERSTANDING
1/2 TSP. OF TESTING
12 OZS. OF TRUST
8 QTS. OF CARING
9 GALS. OF PRIDE
2 PTS. OF MISUNDERSTANDING
AT LEAST 1 HUG DAILY
1 QT. OF ACCOMPLISHMENTS
3 OZS. OF DISAPPOINTMENT
SMILES, FROWNS AND TEARS
MIX TOGETHER WELL AND YOU HAVE PINELAND AS WE KNEW IT.

—A page circulated at Pineland in the 1990s

lives, and care will be forced to decline to the levels of 17 years ago. The state of Maine has always seemed to be a caring state and I can't believe we can't take care of less than 300 retarded people with the quality that we would want any relative to receive."

Critics of the state had learned their lesson in the 1970s. The judicial branch of government would sometimes do what the legislative and administrative branches would not. Perhaps it was time to try again.

Back to Court

In early 1989, the Consumer Advisory Board and its chair, Mickey Boutilier, complained to Susan Parker, commissioner of Mental Health and Mental Retardation, that the state was out of compliance with the decree. Later that year, Parker's replacement, Acting Commissioner Ronald Welch, told reporters that this was apparently so in some areas. The House chairman of the Joint Human Resources Committee also agreed. "They've let this slip," Representative Peter Manning said of state officials in October 1989, "and my view of this is that if they went back into federal court, we would be found in contempt."

"The consent decree establishes a moral as well as legal responsibility," Richard Estabrook, chief advocate in the Department of Mental Health and Retardation, had told the *Maine Times* in 1988. "The state should be willing to enforce it." If the state would not, then the federal court would, he and others believed.

In October 1991, the Consumer Advisory Board moved to test that theory. It filed suit in federal court on behalf of all Pineland residents, naming as defendants Robert Glover, the new commissioner of Mental Health and Mental Retardation; Roger Deshaies, director of the Bureau of Mental Retardation; and Donald L. Hartley, Pineland's superintendent since April 1990.

The state responded that the consent decree had expired. Because Judge Gignoux had "already found the defendants to be in compliance with the terms of

I was the shift supervisor when a guy called up right after the Gulf War. He lived near here, but he had spent time over there. "All the time I was there," he said, "the thing I kept remembering was that Christmas tree at Pineland, the one you see when you drive by. I know it's not Christmas, but could you please light it up anyway?" I called the engineers but we couldn't. All the wiring had just been taken down for the year. I felt so bad for him that we couldn't light that tree.

—*Wayne Haskell, shift supervisor, 2000*

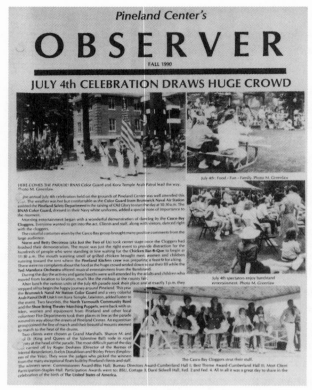

Pineland Center's Observer, *fall 1990 (courtesy of the New Gloucester Historical Society)*

the Consent Judgment," there was no reason for the court to retain jurisdiction indefinitely, Assistant Attorney General Richard Bergeron argued before Judge D. Brock Hornby. Not so, responded Thomas Kelley of Pine Tree Legal Assistance. "We do not think the court dissolved or vacated" the decree, he said.

On April 3, 1992, Hornby found for the state. The decree was no longer valid, he declared. It had expired in 1986, and a new suit would be needed if clients' needs were not being met under federal law.

Parents, employees, union representatives, and community providers who had supported the suit expressed outrage at the ruling. So did Mickey Boutilier. "It's devastating, it's earthshattering," he told the *Lewiston Sun Journal*. "The correspondents are gone. The rights to review aversive programs are gone. . . . We're appealing the decision to the circuit court."

After hearing the case argued in Boston on October 7, 1992, the United States Court of Appeals for the First Circuit ruled that Gignoux had not intended to dismiss the decree, and returned the case to the Portland court, stating as it did that the state was free to file for dismissal. The state did just that, asking the Portland court to terminate the decree as no longer necessary or useful. On September 30, 1993, Judge Gene Carter denied the request. The decree, he said, "has been found by the Court of Appeals for the First Circuit to have created ongoing obligations since it was reached in 1978. Defendants have been unable to make a sufficient showing that changes in factual conditions or law since that time warrant its dissolution." Once again, Pineland and the state must provide services to the standards of the decree or face contempt charges.

"We've been trying to get the Governor and the State to live up to their promises to people with mental retardation for many years," said Boutilier for the Consumer Advisory Board. "Maybe now they will sit down and really talk to us about what needs to be done."

Hearings would soon be under way, and the Carter opinion would have great impact on care given through the end of the century to Maine people with retardation. But it would have less effect on the New Gloucester institution where so many had lived for so long. Pineland's fate was now almost certain. It was closing. The sound and the fury had not yet died out, but the end was coming fast.

In early 1991, the Bureau of Mental Retardation released to media the numbers of people with retardation who were being supported by the Bureau and who were living in or waiting to move into various types of community housing. The facilities are listed in order from most to least restrictive. The first figure in each case shows the number of people in such places; the second shows the number on waiting lists. The word "waiver" refers to Medicare payment arrangements.

    Nursing intensive care facility: 234, 77
    Group intensive care facility: 198, 159
    Waiver boarding homes: 33, 14
    Boarding homes with 15 or more beds: 160, 7
    Boarding homes with 7 to 15 beds: 123, 28
    Boarding homes with 3 to 6 beds: 279, 129
    Waiver foster homes: 400, 127
    Other foster homes: 274, 109
    Living with family: 12, 86
    Supervised living: 20, 134
    Semi-independent living: 50, 69
    Independent living: 368, 62

—Bureau of Mental Retardation

A Decision to Close

The concepts of deinstitutionalization and community care, so important since the 1950s, had largely carried the day by 1990. Pineland's red brick buildings still stood tall in New Gloucester, but water was creeping through the foundations of some, and the lights and heat were off in more.

In 1988, the Bureau of Mental Retardation created a new long-range plan called "A Plan for People." Like the implementation documents that followed, the plan reflected the bureau's continuing commitment to community placement.

No matter how dedicated the staff was to the care of remaining residents, much of its energy still went to helping them move out. "Each new exodus created new expectations for more," Skip Macgowan put it a few years later, and as the departures continued, the in-house caseload decreased faster than expenses did. Some of Pineland's costs were fixed, so annual per resident costs were rising.

"Money had a lot to do with closing Pineland," said Jeff Lee, looking back from the year 2000. He had experienced the center from two directions, first as a resident advocate and later as an administrator and acting superintendent, and he had felt the crunch of need against budget. "It cost a whole lot more to keep people in Pineland than to place them in the community."

Philosophy and practicality also played a part, said Mary Beth Tremblay from the same vantage point. She had visited the center often between 1994 and 1996 as a representative of group homes that were accepting Pineland residents. "I think Pineland just had to close. Once you had the consent decree, you really couldn't apply its concepts to a place like Pineland. It just wouldn't work."

Pressure toward closure was continuing to build in early 1991 when about fifty departmental managers gathered with Commissioner Glover for a retreat at the Bethel Inn. Several years later, Mary Crichton remembered the meeting well. As it opened, Glover was interested in discussing Pineland's possible end but was not yet convinced to push for it. As the meeting concluded, Glover and the rest of his

---

I am angry to think that this entire closure issue is a carefully orchestrated plan meant to keep people in the dark or, at best, to be only partially informed.

I am angry! Parents are frustrated and confused! Staff are angry! Municipal officials are perplexed and deeply concerned!

ENOUGH IS ENOUGH !!!

—*Representative Donnell P. Carroll to Commissioner Robert Glover, December 9, 1991*

> When they stopped using so many restraints, something good began to happen. Behavior got better. People learned to interact with other people in different ways.
>
> —*Nancy Thomas, resident advocate, 2000*

team were sure what they wished to do, even though the current recession would make final community placements difficult.

"We didn't have any bridge money to get us from one point to the other," Crichton said. "But we knew what we had to do, and that was to close Pineland. And after that meeting, there was no turning back. Everybody held their ground."

Was it the right thing to do? Crichton was asked in the year 2000. "Absolutely. No question. This was a good decision."

In early April, Glover disclosed the news to the *Portland Press Herald*. The department's new "policy position," he said, called for placing all Pineland residents in community facilities and closing the center within three to five years. Now the goal was public, if still not widely discussed by state officials and those they served.

Later that year, Roger Deshaies summarized Maine's steps toward closure in a new planning document. The movement had begun more than twenty years before, he said.

> *When the Maine Legislature established the Bureau of Mental Retardation in 1970, the focus of services to persons with mental retardation began to move from the Pineland Center to the towns, cities, and communities throughout Maine. This national movement has essentially been a gradual process of developing community homes and services for both Pineland Center residents and other individuals with mental retardation already living in the community.*

The consent decree and the creation of Medicaid-funded community residence programs were later spurs to the process. New flexibility in federal funding, announced in September 1991, was especially important, because it extended an earlier waiver program and allowed money for community residential training, day care, rehabilitation care, personal support, respite care, crisis intervention, transportation, adaptive aids, communication aids, daily living skills training, supported employment, and environmental modification—in short, the services that Pineland was providing. So the time for change had come. Now the state could close the center and still assist people with retardation, according to the plan:

People are making the transition from Pineland Center to community living:

- Andrea now lives in her own apartment and works. She talks with considerable pride about her apartment and how her quality of living has so improved.

- Elizabeth has lived at Pineland for the majority of her life. Elizabeth requires considerable assistance to manage the many aspects of day to day living. Elizabeth now lives in the community and her mother expresses her appreciation for the realization of a dream nearly fifteen years in the making.

- Fran came to Pineland from an out of state residence. Fran is now a senior in high school, living in a foster home, and a proud member of the local community.

- Bob has lived at Pineland for twenty-five years. Bob has for the past twelve months lived in a foster home, closer to his family.

- Ray has gone home to live with his parents.

The names of the people have been changed but their experiences are real. They represent a small sampling of the successes being experienced by people making the transition from Pineland Center to community living. They stand as examples of people returning to become members of our, and not their, communities. They remind us to guard against underestimating the capabilities of people with disabilities.

—*Roger Deshaies in "The Proposed Closure of Pineland Center," February 15, 1993*

The Department will in no way abandon its commitment and obligation to provide the crisis intervention and support services which Pineland Center has historically provided as the option of "last resort."

In fact, thanks in part to the new Medicaid rules, the decision to close was rapidly becoming action, the *Press Herald* said on February 5, 1992:

Without making a formal announcement, state officials have begun phasing out Pineland Center, Maine's only institution for the mentally retarded.

Twelve of Pineland's 260 mentally retarded residents have been moved to private apartments and houses throughout the state in the past five months.

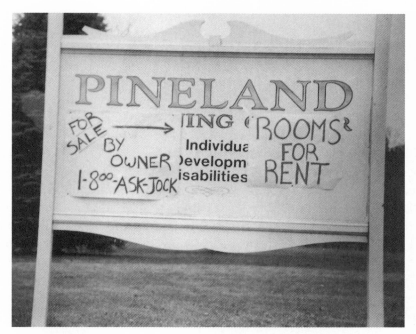

Rooms for rent at Pineland—an anonymous message; "Jock" was the nick-name of Governor John R. McKernan, Jr. (courtesy of the New Gloucester Historical Society)

Deshaies hoped to close the center by the end of 1994, the article continued. Ronald Welch, an assistant commissioner, acknowledged that officials had never formally told families or the public about the closing. "We prefer to talk about new and innovative ways for supportive living approaches in the community, which may and will result in the closing of Pineland," he said.

If defenders of Pineland had envisioned a fight for life from Superintendent Hartley, they were disappointed. "I participated in and supported the discussions which led to the recently announced policy position," he said in the spring 1991 edition of the *Observer*. Pineland's purpose had changed, he added; it had become a "safety net for failed community placements," and a place for crisis intervention best provided elsewhere.

> *[T]he shift from an institutionally-based to a community-based sys-tem has stalled; but not because the vision was wrong, or because the effort by the Department, Bureau, providers and families lacked will and deter-mination! The effort came to a halt because the commitment to fund and sustain it evaporated. The challenges are clear. How do we get things mov-ing again?*

Sound and Fury

In the winter and spring of 1992, the movement to closure advanced dramatically as various parties tried a range of responses to Hartley's question. The Bureau of Mental Retardation held public forums throughout the state in February to discuss its plans. Legislators prepared to consider proposals for diverting some of Pineland's $24 million budget into community services. The result would mean a saving of funds, Governor McKernan had said in November.

There was little consensus about the economics of Pineland and its closing. Some officials argued that annual costs at Pineland per resident were $90,000, whereas similar services could be found in the community for $60,000. Others debated these numbers, and even some community service providers argued that state officials were naive to think that community care would be less expensive than Pineland's. Roger Deshaies publicly disagreed with the governor, saying that the Bureau of Mental Retardation had no evidence the shutdown would mean savings. "We're looking at things being a wash," he said. Anyway, talking about finances "has put the discussion at a wrong place. Closing Pineland is not a financial piece. It is a humanity piece."

Some former supporters of Pineland agreed with his assessment. Reverend Booth, a Pineland parent who had recently completed his term as chair of the Board of Visitors, was among them. The consent decree had called for the development of new community services, he said, and relying on Pineland had hindered that.

But other parents were furious with the state. One was Joan Collins, a member of Pineland Parents and Friends. "The state is telling us that they are giving our children the right to advocate for themselves in the community," she objected. "How can you expect someone with the mental age of two to do that? Some of them can't even talk."

Another was Pauline T. Gelinas, whose son had left Pineland in the early 1980s and returned after a very bad experience. She spoke of the experience in a letter to the editor of the *Lewiston Sun Journal*:

> Your vision is my nightmare. I'm pleading for my son to remain at Pineland.
>
> —*Pauline Gelinas of Mechanic Falls to state officials at a hearing of the legislative Human Resources Committee on February 6, 1992*

While critics of Pineland argue that it is too restrictive (how they love that word) an environment, from my son's perspective it is the exact opposite. You see, he had a taste of group-home living and it nearly destroyed him.

My son cannot function in a community outside Pineland. As seen through his eyes, the larger world is a frightening, confusing, unpredictable environment where he is isolated and in which he has absolutely no hope of ever moving around freely.

At Pineland, his eight-bed home is part of a community with other homes similar to his. He has access to social and medical services, a leisure center, coffee shop, gym and swimming pool—all within an area in which he can safely move around. For my son, it is a safe haven.

"Saying that they belong in the community is just a lot of hogwash," another parent wrote to the editor.

Public meetings of state officials, parents, and the public were sometimes long and loud. "Families, staffers blast plan to close facility," said an early March *Sun Journal* headline above an article describing anger, protest, and tears.

Representative Donnell P. Carroll of Gray frequently joined the fray on the side of the protestors, often speaking for parents, employees, and union members, and sometimes warning of the negative impact that closure could have on the local economy. In late 1992, the state proposed a new "flat-funding budget." Carroll said the move could cost Pineland $28 million in two years and called a news conference at the center's entrance to protest it. "Let's step back, take a deep breath, and see where we are," he said.

State officials told their critics that they would not close Pineland until suitable placements were found for all residents and that they could not close it without legislative approval. But they were now on course and charging rapidly forward. The Bureau of Mental Retardation at this point was serving 4,000 people. It had developed new emergency centers and expanded contracted respite care assistance. It offered crisis services in Presque Isle, Waterville, Portland, Alfred, and Rockland, and it planned to develop more. At the end of November 1992, Pineland's resident population had dropped by another 60 people and stood at 207. The department was including new community services in its request for Medicaid funds. It was considering ways that a community agency could take over the services provided by Freeport Towne Square (a change that would not occur). It was working with a new Consensus Panel appointed by Commissioner Grover. Made up of twenty people representing community agencies, advocates, guardians, parents, and people with retardation, the panel was charged with "working on various aspects of a Pineland cluster plan." It was promoting a new plan for four new community-

> I went to talk with Neville Woodruff once, as a student. I was studying psychiatry at USM, and I said I thought some people needed to be institutionalized. "But young lady," he said, "who gets to decide?"
> —*Mary Beth Tremblay, representative for community group homes, 2000*

based intermediate care nursing facilities with a total of sixty beds that could be used by Pineland residents. And it was still placing Pineland residents elsewhere.

Moving Out

For years, Darla Chafin had visited her daughter at Pineland and taken her for occasional outings. But her daughter's attitude toward the trips began to change as Pineland shrank, remembered Chafin, the president of Pineland Parents and Friends, a few years after the center closed. "She didn't want to get into the car. Too many people were getting into cars and not coming back. And she always wanted to come back."

Through 1992 and beyond, almost everyone at Pineland was highly conscious of the cars that left and did not come back. How they saw the process depended on their perspective. Lewiston's *Sunday* paper showed one viewpoint on February 9, 1992:

> *Patients at Pineland Center for the retarded are "for sale," distraught staffers say.*
>
> *In an escalating controversy over state plans to shut the facility down, workers there claim people are essentially coming in, selecting which patients they think they can handle, and trying to walk off with them.*
>
> *The average Pineland resident has a "price tag" of $56,900, the amount of state and federal funding provided per year of care. Severely retarded and disabled go for more.*
>
> *"It's like slavery," stated former Pineland Mental Retardation Supervisor Diane Haile.*

Haile told of three women coming in and looking for a patient to supplement their income and support a house they were unable to sell. Another staffer spoke of a "Let's make a deal mentality," and a third described the scene as a "meat market." The staffer added, "You work so hard to give clients a little bit of dignity. They didn't ask for this."

Many staff members felt they were losing friends as residents left, friends they might never see again. This could be hard for outsiders to understand in the case

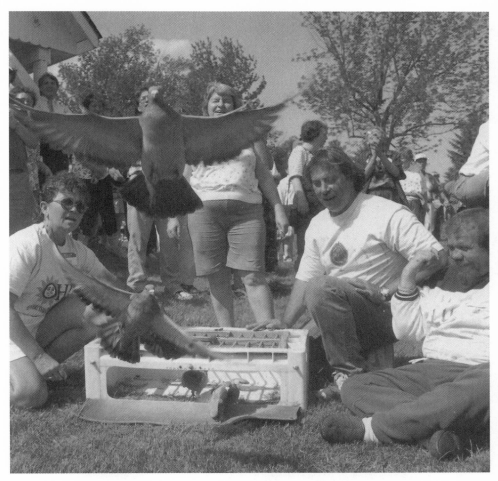

Pigeons flying free at Pineland's closing (courtesy of Ellie Fellers)

of residents who couldn't even speak, the staffers allowed. But working with severely retarded adults is in some ways like dealing with a baby. Maybe they can't talk, was the common explanation, but you can hear them and see them and feel them, and you know what they are telling you. You know what their needs are. But you might not be sure that their needs will be understood and met in their new community setting.

Elaine Gallant was particularly concerned about a woman she had walked with on the grounds of Pineland almost daily. The woman went to a new home in Portland. "Where would she walk in the city?" Gallant asked. "How could that be good for her?"

[These] aren't new ideas, and they aren't my ideas, you've heard them before. But they continually recur to me as I think about and read about the many "programs" we use to "manage" difficult client behavior. Do these assumptions sound radical?

Assumption #1: The assaultive, aggressive, or "acting out" behavior we see in some of our residents has causes. There are reasons that people, even people with mental retardation, behave as they do.

Assumption #2: The "causes" are found in the environment, i.e., the behavior is related to the actions of other people, other clients and staff, and to the ways in which we structure a client's day.

Assumption #3: Aggressive behavior is purposeful, planful, and serves a function for the resident; it is not a random event.

Assumption #4: It is useful to speculate about why the resident behaves as he does because it leads to ideas about what kind of a program might work to eliminate the aggressive behavior.

Assumption #5: "Programs" which address only the question, What do we do (to the resident) when the behavior occurs?, e.g., restraint, time-out, sitting technique, etc, are not programs aimed at the reasons (causes) for the behavior, they are programs for us! They are for our convenience and they represent "standing orders."

As you've probably heard, I think we use too many of these aversive techniques. I'm hoping that some of you will agree with me and work toward their elimination. The question that most frequently is asked in this connection is what other techniques can we use to prevent injury when the resident behaves like this.

Is it worthwhile to redirect our energies toward finding the causes for the behavior and changing them? For example, if Betty goes wild whenever you insist she do something, why insist?

—*Superintendent Donald L. Hartley, Ph.D., in*
"Communicator: Biweekly Bulletin for Staff and
Residents of Pineland Center"

Mary Beth Tremblay saw things differently as she represented group homes eager to receive Pineland clients. She saw more strengths in group homes than in Pineland's piecemeal institutional approach. "You've got your physical therapy and your occupational therapy and your other psychological therapy at Pineland, but they don't connect to each other."

She also saw problems in the treatment of individual residents. "There was one women who I thought really needed to get out of there. I almost put her in the trunk of my car and drove away."

Tremblay also sympathized with Pineland workers. "They weren't just losing friends. They were losing their jobs. A lot of them gave their whole lives there and honestly felt this was the best way to help others."

The departure of Pineland residents was hardly an isolated event. People with mental illness as well as those with mental retardation were leaving institutions all around the nation, and in many cases the moves appeared to be beneficial. But in Pineland's case, parents and residents were sometimes concerned with failed past promises. "Parents' fear is a rational fear, based on their own experiences with the system," Richard Estabrook told the *Sun Journal.* "Promises have been made in the past and they have not been kept. I certainly understand where they're coming from."

"It's hard, parents are scared," added Laurie Kimball, staff advocate for the Consumer Advisory Board. "But all the research and all the studies are saying that if you put these people in their own home and find them a job, they're going to thrive and become part of the community."

Press Reports

News reporters in the early 1990s sometimes followed the fortunes of Pineland clients who had left the center, and not all their stories made it easy to accept reassurances about community placements.

In the fall of 1992, the *Press Herald* told the story of one man who had lived at Pineland for ten years, then moved to Portland, where social workers assisted him at his request but otherwise let him do what he wanted. Life on the client's own terms, said the *Press Herald,* had meant "to buy and use drugs, engage in prostitution daily, beg merchants for handouts or shoplift from their stores, and to rummage through garbage for junk to sell or food to eat."

Retardation officials called this transition a success, the *Press Herald* reported, but Portland's police chief, Michael J. Chitwood, disagreed. "It's a total disgrace the state is putting [the mentally disabled] out there without the resources. It's a tragedy waiting to happen," he asserted.

Another former Pineland resident made the news when a fisherman found him sunburned, dehydrated, and alone, floating in a small boat in the Gulf of Mexico, several miles off the coast. He had apparently gone to Florida because he wanted to see a space launch. How he got to the boat and how long he stayed in it no one knew.

These clients are like my children. I love them . . . You know the most that anybody can know about them . . . I've written eulogies for their funerals. Some of us have been pallbearers.

—*Bliss Hall worker Annette Lausier, to the* Press Herald, *October 3, 1994*

Stories like those might give any parent pause, but more positive reports also appeared from time to time. On July 16, 1995, the *Maine Sunday Telegram* told the story of Frederick Giguere, an eighty-five-year-old man. From the age of four, Fred displayed bad temper tantrums and other behavioral problems. When things grew worse, in 1920, his parents sent him off to the Maine School for Feeble-Minded. Two years later, at the age of eleven, the boy lost all contact with his family. Giguere lived through the farm years of the school and the era of overcrowding, with rooms full of cots and uniforms of V necks and blue pants in a single size with an elastic waist. He lived through the fires and the Bowman reforms and the consent decree and the first years of deinstitutionalization. He lived through it all, and most of the time he lived alone, sticking to himself as much as he could. He did not like rides away from Pineland, and he did not like change. When his dormitory closed in the 1970s, Giguere remained in it anyway for three whole days before the staff could get him to move.

In the 1980s, Giguere met Dennis Hawkes, supervisor of his unit. Hawkes liked the aging resident and worked with him, eventually convincing him to do more, to move further. Fred also met Hawkes's wife, Sharon, who volunteered to be his correspondent and help her husband be sure "the system didn't jerk Fred around," as Dennis put it. Then Giguere met Elaine Gallant, and she became closer to him than anybody else.

With 100 residents left at Pineland, it was time to think of Giguere's move. His supporters put him in a new building to stave off the day. Next they thought about opening a privately run group home on the grounds so he could stay. Then they found a group home in Westbrook where Giguere's Pineland roommate would be.

Pineland staffers took Giguere to visit several times, and they decorated a room to look like his old one. Giguere became angry when Gallant first showed him the room. But later that day he began to accept it. When the staff gave him a choice of two moving dates, he took the first one. A nurse rode with him to the home, and a doctor was on call, but Giguere did not need them. He began instead to settle in, to learn new skills, and to participate more in the life around him. "He just accepted

The Bureau of Mental Retardation currently provides services to nearly four thousand people with mental retardation or autism who live, work, attend school and participate in all aspects of community living. Concerns expressed by some people have centered around the ability to downsize Pineland during a time when resources for people currently living in communities are stretched to their limits.

—*Roger Deshaies in "The Proposed Closure of Pineland Center," February 15, 1993*

everything wonderfully," Hawkes told the *Telegram*. "He blossomed. It made me wonder, Jeez, could it have happened at a different time in his life?"

Nancy L. Thomas, a resident advocate, had summed up such stories in a letter published by the Lewiston *Sunday* on March 1, 1992. "It's a joy to watch people flourish when they move to the community, but that happens only when individual needs are met."

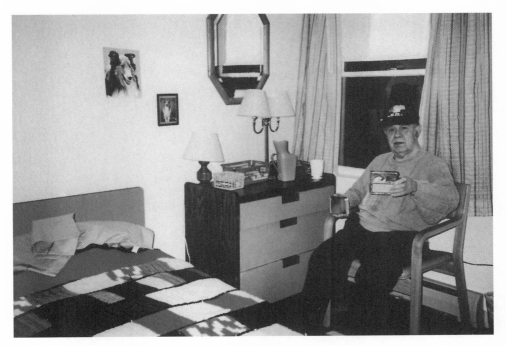

Frederick Giguere in his new room (courtesy of Elaine Gallant)

The Plant

While employees continued their struggles to keep and then replace their jobs, and some parents continued to fight the closing of the institution, others were thinking of the plant itself. With the coming death of Pineland Center, what would happen to the corpse?

When the state decided to close the center, said Representative Carroll, it failed to think about the future of the site, to consider the 650 workers who would eventually lose their jobs, or to include local towns in the planning. That was an oversight the town of New Gloucester intended to correct. In May 1992, its Economic Development Committee asked town manager Bill Cooper to express New Gloucester's interest in helping make future decisions. "We need to direct the decision makers to come up with a master plan so it won't be done hodgepodge," said Cooper.

A few days later the committee toured the plant. State programs active on the campus included the center itself, the regional State Fire Marshal's Office, the canine training program of the Maine State Police, and the Bureau of Intergovernmental Drug Enforcement. Eight major buildings were then idle, with some of them locked to prevent entry and exposure to asbestos. Much of the

POLAND - For 22 summers, mentally handicapped residents of Pineland Center have come to Camp Tall Pines to swim, play and enjoy the outdoors, all courtesy of volunteer workers and donated money.

But the recession is threatening the group that runs the hilltop camp, which sits in the pine woods off Route 26. Donations are down, volunteers are growing scarce, and the group's cash reserves are dwindling.

—Portland Press Herald, *February 5, 1991*

Poland - The cry of a loon echoes across the pond. A stand of tall pine trees shrouds an elegant island home that locals say housed a speakeasy during Prohibition.

Welcome to the magical world of Camp Tall Pines, a picturesque summer retreat established in 1969 on the shore of Lower Range Pond to serve mentally retarded residents of Pineland Center. . . .

A contingent of the camp's former directors gathered at the site Thursday to announce the property and its $65,000 trust fund have been donated to the Maine Special Olympics organization.

—Portland Press Herald, *September 17, 1993*

remaining plant was old and run-down; the power plant alone needed the services of eleven engineers to keep it going around the clock. There were no easy ways to proceed.

In the spring of 1993, officials locked up another building: the Dirigo House, the superintendent's residence through the Bowman era, more recently a home for up to ten people with retardation. An analysis done at about that time showed that closing the remainder of the center would cost the state directly and indirectly some 1,311 jobs, $33.5 million in salaries, and $43.5 million in sales. A year after that, on March 13, 1994, the *Maine Sunday Telegram* presented its readers with a report on the Pineland plant. The thirty-eight buildings on the property contained 490,000 square feet—or eleven-plus acres—of floor space. Once the buildings had housed 1,500 residents; now they held just 140 and provided direct work for 600 employees. Bringing the whole plant up to code would cost $30 million. Even "razing or abandoning the complex would cost millions as well," said the report. New ideas for use mentioned a specialized public school campus and a scientific research institution, but little real planning had yet occurred. Said the *Telegram*:

> *Problems are already evident. A central, antiquated boiler needed emergency repairs for this winter. Water has been unsafe to drink since the compound's treatment plant broke down more than three month ago. Many buildings sit vacant and neglected.*
>
> *"The state has not met its responsibility to keep this facility up for I would say at least 20 years. The whole thing is catching up with us," said Superintendent Paul Peterson.*
>
> *The state's director of planning has proposed a meeting this month among top state officials and local leaders to review possible uses for Pineland. But it may be too late. . . .*
>
> *The physical plant problems and uncertainty are straining a historically friendly relationship with the surrounding community. The Board of Selectmen recently sent a barbed letter to Gov. McKernan criticizing Pineland's deterioration.*
>
> *"We would hope that the planned obsolescence of state facilities . . . is not the accepted norm that your administration will be remembered for," the board wrote.*

Toward the End

By December 1992, Portland officials had become alarmed by the state's projected closing of facilities such as Pineland and the Augusta Mental Health Institute. Mentally challenged people left on their own were endangering themselves and straining local resources. In early 1993, the city filed a class action lawsuit demanding that the state provide basic health care and housing for the mentally disabled.

Many Pineland parents also remained unhappy with the state. They continued to protest Pineland's closing to legislators and reporters, at public and private meetings, wherever they could. But the certainty of the closing seemed to grow every day, and some of the parents showed signs of battle fatigue. "Can you stand another letter regarding the Pineland closing issue?" began a letter to the editor of the *Sun Journal,* a worried complaint from a mother who said her autistic son would need special schooling in Massachusetts if Pineland closed.

Superintended Hartley left Pineland early in 1993. His replacement was Dr. Paul Peterson, a psychologist who had worked at the center on and off since the 1960s. He did not expect his job to be easy. "These are uproarious times here," he told the *Sun Journal.* "There is bad morale and people are in an uproar much of the time."

A year after his appointment at Pineland, Peterson also became a division director in the Department of Mental Health and Mental Retardation. Both his positions made him a target of unhappy parents protesting the transfer of their children to community facilities. Essentially, he told them, former Pineland residents were happier outside the center. Some did have serious problems after leaving the campus, but fewer than 10 of 130 placed in the community had returned. "I'm not saying that we have the first time around met everybody's needs, [but] our success rate is over 90 percent."

Peterson's dual position was not to last long. Melodie Peet, the state's new commissioner of Mental Health and Mental Retardation, fired him and several other top mental workers in what Peterson called the "St. Patrick's Day Massacre" of 1995.

In the meantime, the state had moved even closer to shutting the doors at Pineland. Residents were still moving out, though "no one goes out of Pineland unless the parent or guardian approves," according to Peterson. Guardianship of 600 people was transferred from the state in 1993 to the Maine Advocacy Service of Winthrop, a private group. The move would help the state to avoid conflict of interest when making placements, Peterson explained.

The key to Pineland Center (courtesy of Elaine Gallant)

The *Maine Sunday Telegram* summarized the state's progress for its readers on May 9, 1995, when the resident population had dropped to seventy-six adults. The legislature's Human Resources Committee had decided in March that 1995 would be the year for closure, but Commissioner Peet believed that might be too soon. She appointed a committee of state officials, union representatives, parents, providers, and advocates to consider the timetable. The new panel suggested a six-month delay, with a target date of June 30, 1996. Peet thought even that date might be too early, but she would accept the "logic of the group." The new deadline, she said, was firm.

Saying Good-bye

Maine's press watched carefully as time and departures broke the bonds between Pineland residents and staffers. The *Press Herald* reported on one worker's termination in October 1994:

> *Rachel Beal's layoff notice came this week, and like any layoff in a service business, it means no more paychecks, an end to camaraderie with co-workers and goodbyes to professional clients.*
>
> *Her clients won't return the goodbyes. The people she cares for at Pineland Center have an average developmental age of 6 months. Speech, sign language—sometimes any sign of responsiveness—are beyond them.*
>
> *Yet the slow, inevitable closure of Pineland is breaking bonds between staffers and retarded residents that are as deep as that of parent and child.*
>
> *"It's the same trusting, caring relationship," Beal said. "They know you're going to provide what they need. If I was leaving Bath Iron Works, I'd be leaving a shift. Here, we're leaving people you have relationships with."*

Some connections would continue well beyond the closing. Don Matthews had gone to work at Pineland right after graduating from high school in 1963. He

---

The Fourth of July was a very big day at Pineland. It was a big day for families all over the state. People who had been there before came back to see it again, to see how it had changed.... And it wasn't just the people and buildings that changed. They did, but what changed most was our values. That was the most powerful change, that's what helped close Pineland.

—*Kevin W. Concannon, Maine commissioner of Human Services, looking back in January 2001*

was scared of the clients at first, he remembered. But along the way his attitudes changed, and by 1994 he and his wife, Sharon, a Pineland nurse, were both fond of a thirty-five-year-old resident named Mary. Worried about the care she might receive in the community, they contracted with the state for her care and took her home to join them and their two children as a full-time part of the family. Looking back in the spring of 2001, Matthews reported that the decision had worked out well—"so well that a year later we brought another client into our home."

The Matthews family was not alone. Other Pineland workers made similar arrangements. Still others found new employment in community institutions and continued in that way to work with clients they had known at the center.

In late March 1996, with thirty-one adult residents still at Pineland, Sonya White stood at Pineland talking to a *Press Herald* reporter and trying to remember which darkened window had been her daughter's when she arrived in 1969. "For 23 years my daughter lived here," she said. "I practically lived here . . . It was—it still is such a beautiful campus. It seems so strange. This place is dead."

Not quite, not for another few weeks. Diane Benjamin pushed a wheelchair carrying Pineland's last resident to a waiting van on Monday, May 22, 1996. Ruth Ann had lived at the center for fourteen of her thirty-five years. Now staff members watched her moving away, and reporters watched the whole scene. Ruth Ann seemed "unaware of the change in her life," said the *Press Herald*.

> But staff members were moved as they watched and participated in the symbolic event.
> "It's not easy seeing the place close after so many years. They're like family," Benjamin said of the residents she has worked with for 20 years. "I'm going to be lost without the clients."
> "It's the end of an era. It has a different feel to it," said Eric Gilliam, Pineland's last administrator.

Two months ago, U.S. District Court Judge Gene Carter got so fed up with the lack of an adequate safety net for former Pineland residents that he gave the state until Dec. 30 to develop one—or be held in contempt for shirking its promises in a 1994 class-action suit by advocates for Pineland residents.

Last week, Mental Health Commissioner Melodie Peet unveiled a hastily prepared plan including more than three dozen new workers who will keep track of the 1,100 former Pineland residents scattered across the state.
—*Bill Nemitz*, Portland Press Herald, *December 13, 1995*

"It's a mix of emotions I'm having right now," he said as Ruth Ann prepared to leave.

Closing Ceremony

Pineland's closing ceremony came on a warm, sunny Saturday: June 1, 1996. Dignitaries sat on the bandstand at the front of the grounds, prepared to speak. Other visitors, some in wheelchairs, a number with cameras, moved about the grounds, helping themselves to food, meeting old friends, mixing greetings with good-byes. Those who went to Witham Pond found a new stone beside it, a stone with a plaque and a tribute written by Joan Collins for the Pineland Closure Committee, on which she served: "to all the people who were sheltered here. And to the devoted staff, family and friends who endeavored to make it a home for them."

Many of those people were at the closing, including Ellie Fellers, a former Pineland physical therapist who was now a reporter covering the event for the Lewiston papers. Several years later she placed the crowd's size at about 1,500. One of its members was Neville Woodruff, the lawyer central to the class action suit of the 1970s. The state had not sent an invitation to Woodruff, but Fellers had stepped outside her reporter's role and asked him to attend. "I thought he should be there," she said. "He was important to the history." Now she watched as Woodruff sat on the lawn observing the proceedings and receiving occasional visits from former residents.

"They expressed their appreciation and happiness to live in Maine's communities now," said Fellers's news report.

Is the state better off with Pineland closed? I always answer "yes," but I qualify that. In an institutional setting you always have somebody looking over your shoulder. In smaller places that might not happen. There isn't necessarily anything wrong, but it's certainly a possibility. Some people say that the retarded don't have as much freedom or as many programs now, and that might be true for some. Some people really blossomed when they left, and for others it didn't work out so well. Generally in the last years a lot of people did a really good job moving people out, and that may be the only reason this succeeded. When it started they used to refer to it as going shopping. Somebody would come into a building and look around and talk to the staff and try to figure out which ones were the best ones to take.

—*Joseph M. Ferri, former Pineland superintendent, 2000*

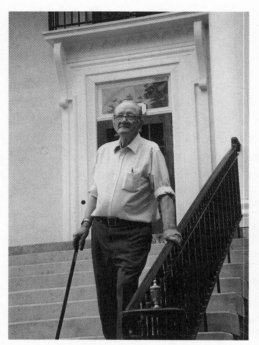

Charles O. Wyman (courtesy of Ellie Fellers)

Governor Angus King's wife, Mary J. Herman, spoke from the bandstand, promising support for people with retardation. "A caring community is a place to be. We are committed to make our communities strong. We will do it in partnership. We will listen every single day. We want to do it right. We're ready to hold hands and work for you."

Wayne Douglas, associate commissioner of the Department of Mental Health and Mental Retardation, also spoke. "This is a happy and bittersweet occasion," he said. "We pause for where we've been and where we're going."

Former residents and other guests received copies of Pineland's master key, the one with the number 709, the one that opened so many doors, the one that symbolized power and freedom. Some of the residents demonstrated their newly granted freedom of choice by moving onto the bandstand stage uninvited and taking over the microphone. This was their story, they said, and they wished to tell it themselves. The assembled dignitaries "never left the stage, but looked dumbfounded and stunned, is my remembrance," Fellers said later.

A one-time resident named Arthur spoke of being on the kitchen staff and confined to the indoors. "I ain't going to come back to this place anymore," he said.

Margaret told of entering Pineland at the age of nine and staying for eleven years. "I've been abused over there, too," she said. "Every time I wet the bed, I got a good spanking by the staff."

Shirley Ware had lived at Pineland from the age of thirteen on into her forties. "I came because I wanted to say my good-by to Pineland for the last time," she said. "I'm glad to see it close. I live in Waterville and have my own apartment, and my dog 'Missy.' I go shopping when I want to."

Charles O. Wyman was there, too, telling again the wonderful story of his escape. He was spending the weekend as an indoor guest at the farm where he had slept in the barn after running away from the school.

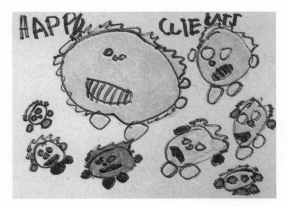

Happy clients—the cover for Pineland's closing program, illustrated by House #1, Freeport Towne Square (courtesy of Elaine Gallant)

A high point in the celebration came with the opening of a cage that contained twelve homing pigeons, the opening and release that signified freedom. Photographers clustered to capture the birds' flight on film, making the images that would be central to the following day's newspaper accounts of the closing.

For this one more day, Pineland's campus was filled again with human sound, with excitement and pleasure, with laughter and speech, with anger and hope, with sorrow and tears.

Some cried with pleasure at the closing of the place, and some cried with fear for their tomorrow. Some cried with relief that the long years of conflict were done, and some cried for friendships lost.

Across the wide lawns, Elaine Gallant watched a senior official walking slowly away from the crowd and the bandstand, his head bent, his face wet with tears.

Gallant was there to assist a client as well as to experience this final Pineland event. She thought she saw her own sadness reflected in the faces of coworkers. She resented the views that some people had of the place where she had worked so many years, and she regretted Pineland's closing.

"We had made a wonderful place there," she said later. "But nobody noticed."

Frederick "Freddie" Giguere, 88, a 75-year resident of Pineland Center who enjoyed watching construction projects and airplane take-offs and landings, died Saturday at a Portland hospital after a brief illness . . .

Mr. Giguere was Pineland's oldest resident at the time the state ordered the institution closed. In April 1995 he moved from the facility to a group home in Westbrook. . . .

Some Pineland staffers were concerned that Mr. Giguere would not be able to make the transition out of the place he considered his home for 75 years.

"He was a quiet, gentle man who had the reputation of being a recluse," said Elizabeth Karlonas, program support coordinator for the group home where he lived.

At Pineland, Mr. Giguere had flatly refused to get into a vehicle. The staff surmised that he did not want to leave Pineland because he was afraid he would not return. They had to give him drugs before they could transport him to the dentist or doctor, according to old Pineland records.

To the surprise of many, Mr. Giguere adjusted to living in a group home in Westbrook. "It was his house and he let everyone know that," Karlonas said. . . .

In Westbrook, Mr. Giguere took an interest in getting out into the community, and learned to make choices in the way he lived. There were several activities he enjoyed, thanks to the support and encouragement of the workers at the group home.

Every day he went to Dunkin Donuts on Main Street for tea and doughnuts. He also enjoyed trips to construction sites to watch the workers and note their progress, visits to the airport to watch the planes, and shopping for clothes and items for his room.

Whenever he left the home he always reminded people that it was his home and that he would be "right here, my home," Karlonas said.

Mr. Giguere enjoyed sanding furniture, tidying up, watching Lassie movies and shuffling around in the kitchen during the late night hours, according to workers at the group home.

He was described as a proud man with a great sense of humor. He never left his room until it was tidy, made sure his hair was combed underneath his baseball cap, and didn't like to acknowledge when he wasn't feeling quite up to par. . . .

There are no known relatives surviving, but Mr. Giguere does leave a loving group of friends that have been his family through the years . . .

—*Will Bartlett*, Portland Press Herald, *July 21, 1998*

Part Three

Preparing for the Future

———

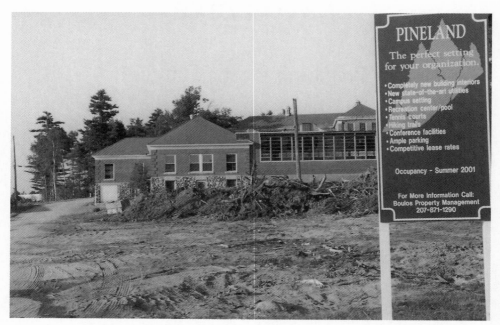

An invitation to the new Pineland (author photo)

Respite and Rebirth: 1996–2000 8

Never think you've seen the last of anything.
—Eudora Welty

Drivers sometimes shivered when they passed the empty Pineland Center on dark winter nights, sensed the hulking shells of cold, crumbling brick, and wondered at their memories. Visitors strolling the grounds by light of day sometimes paused to assess the doubtful potential of the place and ask what could grow out of its moldy decay. Pilots sometimes circled in small planes as they strained to see what remained beneath the pine canopy that cast deep shadows on much of the campus.

Others took more active interest. Among them were those wishing to find new uses for the plant.

Real and Potential New Uses

What should happen to Pineland? And what could happen? Governor Angus S. King, Jr., appointed a Governor's Task Force on Pineland Center Reuse in December 1994. Chaired by Lawrence Zuckerman of New Gloucester, the group suggested a year later that the state refurbish and sell the property piece by piece, because this would cost less than demolishing the buildings and disposing of the asbestos they contained. The King administration balked at the idea of spending millions either way, and determined to try to sell the whole thing as is.

The Pineland Conversion Committee, a state and local group chaired by Charles Jacobs, deputy commissioner of Maine's Bureau of Finance and Administrative Services, then took on the task of marketing the property nationwide, initially with the help of Questor, a Portland-based real estate firm. In 1996, Questor put together an information packet more than six inches thick and asked prospective developers to show how they would handle the property, create jobs,

> I thought there's nothing to be ashamed of in terms of what Pineland was for many years. It was a wonderful farm operation and it was a wonderful facility. Why should all of us shrink from that because of something all of us neglected for a certain period of time? We all do things that are bad. We don't necessarily try to escape from it. It's part of us. . . . We set out very early not to abandon the history. The history is good. We think it is a history that ought to be acknowledged.
>
> —*Owen Wells, 2000*

and contribute to the local economy. There was significant interest; Questor sold ten of its packets for seventy-five dollars each. But a fall deadline passed with no offers made.

Along the way, word somehow got out that landscape architect Frederick Law Olmsted, famous for designing New York City's Central Park, had planned Pineland's core campus. Not so, responded Eleanor Ames and Linda Murnik of the Maine Olmsted Alliance for Parks and Landscapes. The Olmsted firm had been consulted in the early 1920s, but Olmsted himself had died years before. Olmsted was often falsely credited for specific work, Ames told the *Press Herald*. In fact, people also thought that Olmsted had designed a park in Portland. "It drives me, personally, nuts," said Ames.

Also along the way, interest developed in specific pieces of the property. Governor King started some of it when he suggested that Pineland's chapel might be sent south to assist needy victims who had lost their own building to arson. Wait a moment, responded some Maine congregations. We could use a building, too. But the chapel lacked a full foundation. Moving it would be difficult, and it remained on its slab.

Interest in the old infirmary—Perry Hayden Hall—proved more fruitful. On September 26, 1998, after several years of negotiating and planning at the state and local levels, School Administrative District 15, serving Gray and New Gloucester, rededicated the structure as the Burchard A. Dunn School and filled it

> When I drove through Pineland last week, its empty buildings were ghostly in the morning fog. Rows and rows of windows have gone dark. Oversized swings and dilapidated merry-go-rounds stand unmoving under the trees.
>
> —*Roberta Scruggs,* Maine Sunday Telegram, *April 28, 1996*

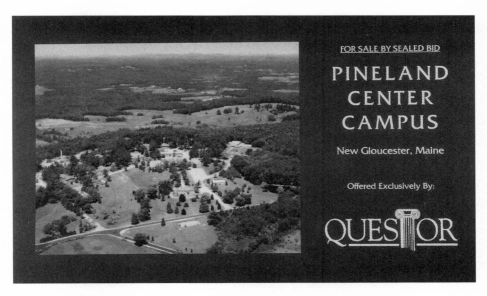

Questor's Pineland offering (courtesy of Elaine Gallant)

with 400 elementary school students and their teachers. The old infirmary's location across Morse Road from the central campus made it a good choice for the district. "It rocks," a seven year old told a reporter who asked his opinion of the new school. "The gym is awesome. We get to do relay races."

The Conversion Committee, in the meantime, had set a new deadline of April 4, 1997, for proposals. Its members expected that they might receive none, in which case the committee would be replaced by a development authority. But two offers and a letter of interest arrived before the deadline. The most appealing of the three came from the Liberty Group, a Portland-based firm that proposed spending $50 million to develop housing and offices at the center. "The train is leaving the station," said Chairman Jacobs. But the train did not get far. In July, the Liberty Group withdrew its offer. The involved parties disagreed about reasons for the plan's collapse, but environmental concerns, such as the presence of asbestos, were clearly among them.

In February 1998, an Augusta couple proposed a school for special needs students but failed to show access to the necessary financial resources. In October, Platz Associates of Auburn signed a tentative agreement to explore the possibility of renovating the buildings one by one, but that plan, too, soon died. In November 1999, Governor King returned from a trade mission to Taiwan with news of an economic development model he thought might apply to Pineland. But as the end of

All the children are gone now. But their images linger.

Boys and girls. Huddled on floors and beds. Partially clothed. Their frail limbs bound by soiled sheets. Their sallow skin pocked by scabs and lesions from years of self-mutilation.

—Lewiston Sun Journal, *2000*

the century approached, with every rain and every snow advancing the rot of Pineland's buildings, the center's future appeared far from promising. Its neighbors waited on, their hope growing thin as they tried not to dwell on the waste treatment proposal and the prison plan that had once frightened them, or on vaguely possible industrial plans that could destroy the rural character of their towns.

The Continuing Impact of Pineland

Much of the energy devoted to supporting people with retardation had moved from the campus to the many community-based programs and facilities scattered about the state. But Pineland remained key to the effort, because a court-based consent decree continued to set treatment standards for the thousand Pineland residents covered by it. In this fact lay a new problem: 3,500 other Maine people with retardation were not included in the court order. Advocates added concern about creating a two-tier system to their worry about what they judged to be the state's continuing inadequate care of people in both groups.

So the struggles to assist people with retardation went on and seemed likely to persist for years to come. Advocates who had fought to get better programs at Pineland now strove to get them elsewhere. In 1998, state officials asked the federal court in Portland to dissolve its 1994 consent decree. Maine was in compliance, they said, and could do a better job without the court order. That was wrong, responded critics such as Richard Estabrook, the patient advocate for what had become the Department of Mental Health, Mental Retardation and Substance Abuse Services. Eventually the two sides agreed to use an independent auditor to

I will venture a guess that eventually there will be a tendency to reestablish a Pineland.

—*Dr. H. Jay Monroe, former interim superintendent at Pineland, 2000*

resolve their differences. The court assigned New York lawyer Clarence Sundram to assess the state system. In April 2000, Sundram reported back that although many people were making "exemplary efforts" to serve Pineland residents, the state was not providing consistent services or monitoring them as it should. "Maine still fails mentally retarded," announced the *Press Herald*'s front-page headline.

The King administration did not dispute the findings. "I would say that they identified some areas that we need additional work on," said Mental Health commissioner Lynn F. Duby. But, she predicted, the state could probably be in full compliance within a year.

People and Things

Pineland was remembered in the late 1990s for more than its impact on other programs. One of its strongest support groups, Pineland Parents and Friends, continued to meet for several years, though it seemed to be faltering a bit at century's end. "Now it's time to think about what we're going to do next," said its president, Darla Chafin, in September 2000.

Most of Pineland's records landed in the Maine State Archives in Augusta. These included 111 boxes of patient case files, superintendents' correspondence, visitors' books and trustees' books, operating room records, annual reports, trustee reports, patient financial ledgers, official notices, discharge ledgers, *Observer*s, and more. Most of the paperwork and other materials the state did not want—several shelves and file drawers full—went to the New Gloucester Historical Society. But another pile of papers had gotten so wet while stored in Yarmouth Hall that it had to be thrown out.

Other physical mementos of the center spread around the state and beyond. Formal paintings of Pineland superintendents went to appropriate family members when they could be located. Keys and some photographs given out at the time of the center's closing found their way into uncounted scrapbooks and drawers. A bronze plaque from the chapel spent the summer of 2000 leaning against Darla Chafin's deck in Augusta, waiting for a more permanent home. The chapel's bell had already gone to a school in Litchfield. And the last pew from the chapel went

---

We're housing the pew here at St. Gregory's in memory of all that went on over there that was good and healthy. Having the pew means that a little piece of the past can go on. It will help young people, especially, to know what was there.

—*Susan W. Austin, Conversion Committee member*

> The state has not met its responsibility to keep this facility up for I would say at least 20 years. The whole thing is catching up with us.
> —*Superintendent Paul Peterson, March 1994*

to St. Gregory's Catholic Church in Gray, its release for the purpose negotiated by Susan W. Austin, Gray's representative on the Conversion Committee. The church, its parishioners, and its priests had often assisted at the chapel, and Austin wanted to honor their efforts while preserving a part of the past. So she enlisted her husband and a son and together they wrestled the pew onto a trailer attached to their truck and hauled it first to their home, then to St. Gregory's.

Setting a Stone

When they gathered in May 1996 for their final meeting at the center, members of Pineland Parents and Friends visited Pineland's cemetery and placed flowers at the graves of deceased residents.

The cemetery was also in the thoughts of Elaine Gallant as she began her new career of working in community facilities caring for people with mental disabilities. The quiet memorial grounds on Route 231 held the remains of more than 150 people. They included the former population of Malaga Island, the living and the dead taken from the island by the state in 1911 and 1912, many for incarceration or reburial at the Maine School for Feeble-Minded. Gallant had seen the several memorial stones bearing only names and the single date of 1912, and regretted that they failed to explain the similarity of the dates or give visitors any hint of the story they represented. So she did something about it.

Once the state had transferred ownership of the cemetery to the New Gloucester Cemetery Association, Gallant requested and received permission to place a new marker. Using money of her own and contributions from her family and the North Yarmouth Historical Society, she ordered a large stone marker with a simple rowboat carved near the top and these words: "Nov. 1912. The people living on Malaga Island, New Meadows River, Maine were relocated." Then on a cold, rainy day, Gallant, her brother, and a friend of his moved the marker into place. The strange, sad tale of Maine's attempt to purify its coastal real estate by forcibly removing its inhabitants was now plainly but forever marked in stone.

Remembering Pineland

The news media remembered Pineland, too. Portland, Lewiston, and other newspapers frequently reported on attempts to sell and rejuvenate the campus, and occasionally told stories of Pineland's past. Diane Atwood, a television reporter for Portland's WCSH, took a special interest, interviewing Charles O. Wyman and others, leading them to share their memories of Pineland with viewers. "I really got caught up in delving into Pineland's history," Atwood said early in 2000. "I've done four stories so far, and plan to do one or two more in the near future on the consent decree and some of the last people to leave. My grand plan is to produce a one-half hour documentary."

Atwood's reporting had an impact beyond what she might reasonably have expected, because it caught the attention of a man whose vision would eventually transform Pineland. He was Owen W. Wells, president of Portland's Libra Foundation.

A New Idea

Elizabeth B. Noyce, whose former husband had made a fortune as a computer pioneer and a founder of the Intel Corporation, created the Libra Foundation in 1989 to help fund charitable "organizations, activities, operations or purposes" within the state of Maine. When Noyce died in 1996, Wells, her attorney, friend, and advisor, became Libra's president.

By the late 1990s, Libra's impact on Maine was extensive and expanding fast. It had built a new indoor public market on Portland's peninsula, and it had made many grants large and small—ranging from $5,000 to $1 million—for conservation, sports centers, camp scholarships, academic support, and more. It was always on the lookout for new projects, and in December 1999 Wells responded to an Atwood news report by turning his attention to New Gloucester.

"I wonder what's going on with that place," he said, and drove out from Portland to see. Soon his vision grew larger than anything proposed for the property before. Fortunately, Libra's financial resources, placed by the press at more

---

If he is not quite up to the energy level of a kid in a candy shop, he is a far cry from a staid business executive.

"We're going to put the equestrian center right there," he says enthusiastically. And then he launches into a spirited discussion of how riding a horse does so much for not just troubled youths but many of the disabled.

"People in a wheelchair are always looking up at people," he says, scrunching down a bit. Then he rises to his tiptoes. "But on horseback, they not only are higher than the people around them, but they have the joy of riding outdoors, through these magnificent woods, over the fields."

—*The* Portland Business Journal, *speaking of Owen Wells, 2000*

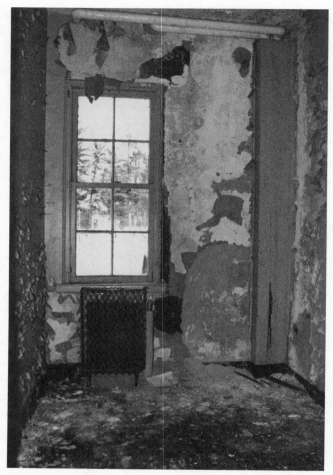

Interior of Yarmouth Hall, January 2000 (author photo)

than $300 million, were already more than large enough to support the dream—and growing larger with passing time. "Libra anticipates its assets will continue growing during the new year to a point that will eventually make it one of the wealthiest foundations in the U.S.," Wells told colleagues in a report on the year 1999. "Obviously, this will create an opportunity for consideration of more grants to more deserving nonprofit organizations in Maine than previously imagined."

But Wells and Libra had more than vision and money on their side. They also had the flexibility and quick punch of a small, focused organization, a combination to boggle the mind and stir the envy of any state bureaucrat. Wells could convert thought into action with remarkable speed, and in this case he did. On

Thursday, December 30, he shared his vision at a public meeting of the Pineland Conversion Committee.

"What a tragedy," he said. "All those buildings—wonderful buildings—all going to waste." But not for long. Wells spoke of a therapeutic riding program, commercial greenhouses and restored farms, call centers and new care for people with physical and mental challenges, rural trails and recreation, commuter trains that could run from Portland to Pineland.

New Gloucester selectman Matthew Sturgis told Wells that his plan was a Christmas present to the town. "Thank you for offering up this kind of opportunity," he said.

A New Pineland

Early in 2000, Wells traveled frequently out and about the Pineland neighborhood. Stopping at a local bakery, he asked if owners would wish to relocate to Pineland. Lunching at a favorite restaurant, he wondered if its owners would consider the Pineland setting. He already knew that Maine Bank & Trust would probably have a branch there. That was a logical step; Elizabeth Noyce had founded the bank.

The new Pineland plans specifically included people with disabilities. They could and should be integrated there the way they should be integrated into the larger community, said Wells. Accomplishing that, Pineland could make itself a model for the rest of the country. Between 150 and 200 Maine youths were being treated out of state because Maine lacked facilities, Wells said, his argument reminiscent of the reasons given for creating Pineland as the Maine School for Feeble-Minded in 1908. The cost to the state for such care was in the millions. "If you are going to spend it, why not spend it in Maine?"

With winter moving into spring, new life was occasionally apparent in various buildings. Engineers checked asbestos and safety, planners decided what should go and what should stay, reporters and photographers took fresh looks, and laborers dropped limbs and trees damaged by time and ice storms. Tentative ideas began emerging in the form of more specific plans for a therapeutic riding stable, recre-

> Jaws hit the floor in New Gloucester last December . . . when Mr. Wells visited and told town leaders he was interested in buying the 1,000-acre mental-health campus after seeing it mentioned on television. "We all kind of sat there with our chins down," says Steve Libby, chairman of the New Gloucester planning board. "We considered it a big Christmas present."
> —*The* Wall Street Journal, *June 7, 2000*

A considerable amount of time was spent on the eventual sale of Pineland Hospital to the Libra Corporation, a non-profit foundation established by the late Betty Noyce. Although this property is in New Gloucester, whatever happens there will affect both towns in, I believe, a positive way. To begin with, the expense of $250,000 each year to watch it fall apart was eliminated.
—*Clifton E. Foster, state representative for Gray and New Gloucester, in the* New Gloucester News

ational trails and tennis courts, and a visitors' center where people could climb onto a horse-drawn carriage to tour and see cattle grazing and gardens producing food around the calendar.

At times so much was happening on the campus that visitors might have been surprised to learn that Libra and the state had not yet come to terms on a property transfer. That, too, was in the works. The October Corporation, an operational arm of Libra, and Boulos Property Management, a real estate firm, were central to the negotiations. Libra wanted not just the central Pineland campus but some of the surrounding state grounds as well. When this proved a stumbling block in February, negotiations faltered and Libra pulled most of its people from the project. But Wells and Governor King each gave a push and the process moved forward again, slowly at first, then accelerating at a remarkable rate.

In July the deal was done, and papers were signed. Libra agreed to pay the state $200,000 for the campus itself and $540,000 more for 617 acres around it. It expected to spend $40 million fixing up the place, and more adding bits and pieces of property around the edges.

Soon a large power shovel moved into place and took its first bites from the roof of the chapel, an early victim of the change. Bishop Hall came down, and new tennis courts appeared in its place. The Federation Village, the carpentry building, the fire station, Longley Center, and Sebago House all came down. So did numerous trees. To viewers on surrounding hills, Pineland seemed to be emerging from under the pine canopy that had hidden it away for years, its remaining buildings now reaching up and out instead of crumbling down. To viewers on the grounds, the distant peaks of the White Mountains appeared more frequently, and the sun offered longer moments of warmth and light.

Commuters passing the campus could never be sure what they would see the next time they came by or what the result of all the commotion would be. They could only be sure that almost every day when they passed, almost every day for the next few years, they would see change.

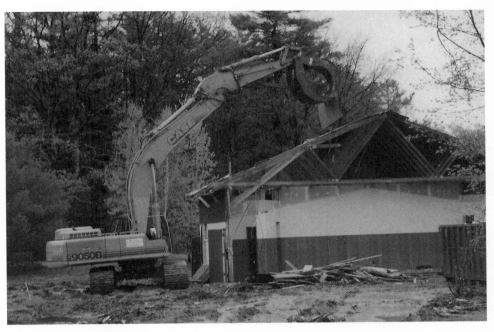

Chapel coming down (author photo)

Journalists seemed to be generally impressed, if sometimes startled, by the quick transition. "I had lunch the other day with Owen Wells, just the two of us," wrote the editor of *The Portland Business Journal* in an article with more than 1,600 words describing a trip to Pineland in a pronounced "gee-whiz" tone. "It was a mighty interesting day."

There were critics and skeptics, of course. Some wondered if people with retardation or other challenges would wish to be on a campus so far from an urban setting or in a place with a name that had once signified confinement. Some were

> We need to ask what happens if society doesn't value you. . . . If we look at Pineland's history carefully, we can learn a lot about ourselves. . . . If we really look at what happened, and if we're honest, maybe we can do better for all of us.
>
> *—Mary Beth Tremblay, representative for community group homes, 2000 annual report, July 1, 1999–June 30, 2000*

troubled by thoughts of new traffic and pressure on local housing and schools. Some scoffed at the idea of providing train service.

But by late 2000, actual change was fast outpacing doubt. Two eighty-nine year olds, at least, were very pleased, they told the *Sun Journal*. "I think it's a wonderful thing to have them make use of the place like that," said Louisa Bishop, the daughter of Pineland's first head farmer. "There was a lot of sadness about that place just sitting there."

Charlie O. Wyman, Pineland's renowned escapee, agreed. "I think that's a very good thing," he said. "It's a beautiful place there. It could be used for something very important."

Afterword

It is not the literal past, the "facts" of history, that shape us, but images of the past embodied in language.
                                                            —Brian Friel

What will tomorrow's Pineland be? We cannot know. The future always dawns as a question mark.

Ellie Fellers, a longtime Pineland observer and an early reader of this book, is confident that tomorrow will at least be good. "Libra will succeed," she concluded as she waxed poetic in the earliest hours of a day deep in November 2000. "The battered bride Pineland has found a suitor worthy to restore her tattered exterior, give her heart a lift and thrust her ahead for a new mission."

I watch with wonder and hope on my frequent trips past the changing campus. Then my mind turns away from tomorrow and back to the past to wrestle with its unanswered questions. I expect I will not escape this backward draw until *Pineland's Past* is in print.

I knew when I began work on the book that it would not be Pineland's definitive history, and questions would remain at its completion. I preferred to use the time and other resources at my disposal to paint an anecdotal picture, not to build a dry and unassailable structure of statistic and fact. I intended to rely on secondary sources, too, and treat things such as contemporary news reports as informative parts of the story. But when I began to fill in the gaps by speaking with participants in the Pineland story, I found it hard to stop. Each person I approached had informative things to say and more people to suggest for interviews. As deadlines closed in and I ended the process, I knew that I would not only fail to answer all my questions but could not stop asking more.

A few of my continuing questions appear below. I present them in the hope that future studies of Pineland will help to complete my partial and tentative answers.

How many lives did Pineland help shape?

During my research I asked Maine's Department of Mental Health, Mental Retardation and Substance Abuse Services how many residents Pineland had served through the years. Two days later a representative politely suggested that I dig through the archives to find my own answer. Time did not allow me to take on the thankless task of sifting through box after box of dusty records. I went back instead to the sixty-year anniversary edition of the *Pineland Observer*, which said in 1968 that "almost 4,400 persons have been residents, patients if you will, and many more are still to come." Assuming the accuracy of that figure and extrapolating ahead through the next thirty years while remembering the declining population, one can comfortably add another 2,000 and come up with a working total of 6,400 residents.

But that figure does not include nearly all of the people whom Pineland touched, often deeply. There were many employees, too, 600 at one point in 1994, thousands through the years. Add to that the families of residents and sometimes employees as well. The decision to place (or not place) a person in Pineland could have profound impact on parents and siblings alike. Then there were temporary users; they included occasional patients at Hedin Hospital beginning in 1931 and many others who came in later years for diagnosis, training, treatment, and respite—2,000 in 1980 alone.

How many lives did Pineland help shape? The answer is probably in the lower tens of thousands. I decided at one point on 25,000 as a useful starting point for discussion. When I mentioned that number to Kevin W. Concannon, commissioner of Maine's Department of Human Services, he replied that it seemed high and suggested 20,000 instead. So now I offer a range of 20,000 to 25,000. If other researchers ever attempt more exact counts, I'll be fascinated to see their conclusions.

What are the lessons of Pineland?

The story of Pineland offers many lessons, and I hope that readers can find them in this book without my rising to a soapbox and preaching. But one of those lessons raises enough guilt and concern in me that I wish to pronounce and share it here: We who are not directly involved with social and health institutions such as Pineland must not simply turn them over to either state or private agencies and assume that all is well. We should watch the news reports and react to what is bad and what is good. We should take a direct interest and we should sometimes visit when invitations are extended—and maybe also when they are not. We should do this now, just as we should have done it during Pineland's day.

I have lived in Maine almost all my life, and within easy reach of Pineland for more than three decades. Pineland was partly mine until its sale in 2000. As a citizen of Maine I owned it. My taxes supported it and my attitude failed it. I certainly read from time to time of open houses and other opportunities to find out more about the institution. But I took no real interest in it until after it had closed. Mea culpa. Had I done more, had I visited and maybe volunteered, I might have helped improve it. I certainly would have come to understand and appreciate its residents and staff long before they went away.

Was Pineland an abusive or a comforting place to be?

It was either and it was both. Some residents received warm, loving care. Others knew mistreatment.

Abusive behavior grabs the attention of the casual observer. People read news reports about the misbehavior of the few and remark on that without recognizing the nurturing efforts of the many. They conclude that places such as Pineland are as bad as the worst they have heard. But the Pineland of the past was much more than the sum of its problems; it was also the source of much good.

Pineland's senior administrators were generally alert to the possibilities of mistreatment and ready to fire or otherwise discipline employees who stepped out of bounds. But definitions of abusive behavior changed through the years, and approaches accepted in the early twentieth century seem wrong to us now. Levels of staffing changed, too, and when staff-patient ratios were at their worst, superintendents could not possibly know of every wrong act committed on the grounds. In later years, with the ratios improving and resident advocates always alert to problems, conditions and treatment became distinctly better.

Nancy Thomas was one of the advocates. "I spent a lot of time seeing the dirty side of Pineland," she recalled in the year 2000. "Still, as institutions go, it was a good institution." Another advocate, Carroll M. "Skip" Macgowan, who started work at Pineland in 1975, offered his own judgment about stories he had heard of earlier abuse in earlier decades, abuse such as ice baths and beatings. "You hear a lot of those stories," he said, "and they are all true."

Possibly, even probably so. If some staff members slipped over the line and abused residents in the 1980s even with advocates on campus watching over their shoulders, surely others abused their charges, sometimes severely, in earlier times when nobody was looking.

But the frequency of such acts can never be known. And acknowledging them in no way denies the extraordinary efforts that other employees sometimes made to improve the lives of their patients and friends. The frequency of these gifts can never be determined either, but they were not unusual. In fact they were common enough to help inspire Ellie Fellers's faith in the future. "The people who lived and worked at Pineland leave a spirit within the mortar and bricks that can never fade," she said.

Was Pineland more a product of its period or its people?

Every investigation into the past must to some degree involve the balance of historical trend and individual contribution. International and national attitudes toward and responses to retardation laid the groundwork for the Maine School for Feeble-Minded, and developments through time and around the world helped determine every major shift in the school's identity.

But the ladies of Portland and the legislators and the first board members and all those who followed were important, too. From the stuff and substance of their era they built a special and distinctive institution.

There were through Pineland's history some very strong persons who had great impact on its development. Dr. Peter W. Bowman is the obvious example. Superintendent in the 1950s and 1960s, he molded Pineland to his own ideals in a way that few others could or would have attempted. Others might have done the job and done it well without building a psychiatric hospital, without bringing a German background to the job and other European doctors to the school, without achieving international acclaim, without fighting so angrily, frequently, and bloodily with Augusta's bureaucrats and politicians.

Was Pineland more a product of its period or its people? I cannot say. People help determine what occurs until critical mass is reached and inevitable force sweeps them all along with it. Swimmers tossed by the tides change the way that waves reach the shore, and people shape their time as it shapes them. Which is in charge? Neither and both. That is the essence of historical change.

Should we honor Pineland's history?

I asked that question as I began the process of creating this book. I decided then, as I have stated in the Preface, that it was possible and right to honor Pineland's past. Now as I conclude the project, I affirm the decision. The story of Pineland is the story of trying, of sometimes failing and sometimes succeeding, but always of trying, sometimes heroically, against excruciating odds. I hope that *Pineland's Past* conveys the energy and essence of this struggle. Yes, we should honor Pineland's history. It is, after all, our own history.

But as Ellie Fellers suggests after decades of watching the Pineland story, we can honor Pineland best if we first heal the wounds left by the struggles of its final years. The key to healing may lie in seeing more clearly what transpired and recognizing the intensity of care exhibited on all sides. Honoring requires acceptance, and acceptance requires understanding. Perhaps this book will help to build that understanding.

Was Pineland good for Maine and its people?

I have asked many individuals to respond to questions such as this, and their answers have varied greatly. Two former administrators indicate the range. One is Dr. H. Jay Monroe, who was acting superintendent for a short time after Bowman left. He would not rebuild Pineland as it was, he made clear in the year 2000. But neither would he apologize for all that Pineland was. Institutions are needed for some people with retardation, he argued. "There are people who need such structural support. It would be nice if everyone was self supportive, but that's not the case."

For Jeff Lee, an assistant superintendent twenty years later, the price of institutionalization was simply too high. "Is Maine better off because Pineland existed?" I asked. "No," he said. "The act of severing an individual's connection with his family and community is just plain wrong."

Other answers fell all across the continuum. One, from Mary Crichton, had the tone of an epitaph ideal for placement here:

> *Pineland did everything bad that every other institution in this country did.*
>
> *It did everything good that every other institution did.*
>
> *Pineland was a product of its time. It needed to be, and it needed to end.*

"Those Who Knew"

"Hate-filled,"
Those who knew said.
And he climbed sleepily into my lap . . .
He buried his tousled head
in my cool green sweatshirt
And wrapped his grubby arms
about my neck . . .

"Uncontrollable,"
Those who knew said.
And he lay quietly beside me
listening to my fairytales
and lullabies . . .

"Refuses to participate,"
Those who knew said.
And he took my hands and
let himself be led into the
midst of dancing and singing . . .

"Will not cooperate,"
Those who knew said.
And he stood beside me
drying the dishes
I had washed . . .

"Will not speak,"
Those who knew said.
And we walked through the forest,
talking of birds
and squirrels and
flowers . . .

"Incapable of love,"
Those who knew said.
And he planted a slobbery
little boy kiss on my cheek . . .

"Hopeless,"
Those who knew said.
And he sang with me
of stars and happiness . . .
He smiled with me at silly jokes . . .
Those who knew . . .
Forgot about love.

—*Julie Parsons, TORCH (Idaho Youth Association for Retarded Citizens) state president, 1970–1971, from the* Pineland Observer, *March 1979*

Chronology

1907 - Legislature votes to establish a school for "idiotic and feeble-minded"
1908 - Maine School for Feeble-Minded created in New Gloucester
George S. Bliss, M.D., named first superintendent
1911 - Gray Hall and Staples Hall constructed
1912 - State removes residents of Malaga Island
Legislature investigates school
Carl J. Hedin, M.D., becomes superintendent
1915 - Nurses' home (Sebago House) constructed
1917 - Central kitchen, dining hall, and bakery built
1919 - New Gloucester Hall opens
Stephen E. Vosburgh, M.D., becomes superintendent
1921 - Yarmouth Hall, powerhouse, and laundry constructed
1925 - Maine School for Feeble-Minded becomes Pownal State School
1926 - Pownal Hall opens
1931 - Hedin Hospital opens
1932 - Department of Health and Welfare assumes responsibility for school
1937 - Cumberland Hall and Vosburgh Hall open
1938 - Nessib S. Kupelian, M.D., becomes superintendent
1944 - Bishop Hall opens
Vocational building opens
1948 - Edward P. Witham, Jr., becomes business agent
1949 - Bliss Hall and Kupelian Hall open
1951 - Maine Federation of Women's Clubs issues critical report
1953 - Peter W. Bowman, M.D., becomes superintendent
1956 - Driver education begins
1957 - Pownal State School becomes Pineland Hospital and Training Center
1958 - Benda wing, Berman School, Federation Village, and new laundry open
1960 - Doris Sidwell Hall dedicated
1961 - Hill Farm closes
Children's Psychiatric Hospital opens

1963 - Full accreditation granted
1965 - Governor Edmund S. Muskie Treatment Building dedicated
       Gym construction begins
1967 - Valley Farm closes
1968 - Benda Hospital, Bliss Vocational Rehabilitation Center open
1969 - Tall Pines Day Camp opens
1970 - All Faiths Chapel dedicated
       Fire station constructed
       Pool added to Soucy gymnasium
1971 - Renovations of Pownal Hall and Kupelian Hall begin
       Patient participation in Special Olympics, Little League begins
1971 - Harry Elizarian becomes acting superintendent
       H. Jay Monroe, Ph.D., becomes acting superintendent
1972 - Conrad R. Wurtz, Ph.D., becomes superintendent
1973 - Children's Psychiatric Hospital closes
       Pineland Hospital and Training Center becomes Pineland Center
1975 - Margaret Bruns becomes acting superintendent
       George A. Zitnay becomes superintendent
       Class action suit filed
       Maintenance building constructed
1976 - Richard Bogh becomes acting superintendent
1977 - Will Burrow becomes superintendent
1978 - Charlene Kinnelly becomes acting superintendent
       Consent decree issued
       New vehicles purchased
1979 - Kevin W. Concannon becomes acting superintendent
       George A. Zitnay becomes superintendent
       Sheltered workshop moves to Freeport Towne Square
1980 - Lincoln Clark replaces David D. Gregory as court master
       Several buildings are renovated
1981 - Court ends supervision of Pineland
       Department of Mental Health and Corrections becomes Department
           of Mental Health and Retardation
1983 - Court ends supervision of community care for former Pineland
           residents
       Berman School closes; programs move to Perry Hayden Hall
1984 - Joseph M. Ferri becomes superintendent
       Behavior Stabilization Unit opens
1986 - Pineland again accredited

Kevin W. Concannon becomes acting superintendent
Spencer Moore, Ed.D., becomes superintendent
1990 - Jeffrey R. (Jeff) Lee becomes acting superintendent
Donald L. Hartley becomes superintendent
1991 - Department of Mental Health and Retardation decides to close
        Pineland
1992 - Federal court in Portland rules for state, against Pineland
Federal Court in Boston overturns Portland decision
1993 - Paul Peterson becomes superintendent
1994 - Governor's Task Force on Pineland Center Reuse forms
1995 - Eric Gilliam becomes chief operating officer
1996 - Pineland closes
2000 - Libra Foundation purchases Pineland plant and land

Index

abuse, allegations of, 75–78, 88, 185–190,
    237. *See also* neglect, allegations
accidents, 38, 67, 71
accreditation, 95, 118, 149, 170, 186, 243
Administration Building, 176
advocacy groups, 125, 162–164
AFL-CIO, 150
All Faiths Chapel, 107, 243. *See also* chapel
almshouses, 3
Altrusa Club, 107
American Association on Mental
    Deficiency, 122
American Federation of of State, County
    and Municipal Employees, 90–91,
    135–136, 140–141
American Psychiatric Association, 94
Ames, Elanor, 224
Anderson, Albert, Jr., 115, 124, 127, 135,
    140, 161
Andrews, J.R., 58
Anspach, Allison, 144–145, 164
apple orchard, 96
Arsenault, Bob, 131
Arthur (resident), 218
attendants, 28
    duties of, 91–92
    under Hedin, 18
    wages of, 116
    See also direct care workers; employees;
        matrons
Atwood, Diane, 228–229
Augusta Mental Health Institute, 213
Augusta State Hospital, 24, 73, 90, 95, 118

Austin, Susan W., 227–228

B., Edward (resident), 58, 60
bakery, 242
Bangor State Hospital, 24, 73, 90, 99, 118
Barrows, Lewis O., 58, 62
Barry, William David, 135
Bartlett, Will, 220
basketball, 123
Bates College, 39, 45
bathing suits, 102
Baxter, Percival, 29–30
Beal, Rachel, 215
behavior modification, 187
Behavior Stabilization Unit, 172, 185,
    187–189, 188, 243
Benda Hospital, 243
Benda wing, 101, 242
Benjamin, Diane, 216
Benoit, Joan, 181
Bergeron, Richard, 198
Berman, Edward J., 90
Berman School, 65, 105, 118, 133,
    177–178, 242, 243
Berry, Clarence, 108
Binet-Simon Test, 16
Bishop, Louisa Lowe, 41–42, 46–47, 48,
    234
Bishop, Neil S., 56, 65–66
Bishop Hall, 66, 232, 242
Bliss, George S., 242
    comments on residents, 8, 9, 12
    first patient and, 6

245

hiring of, 4, 5
plans of, 10–13
Bliss Hall, 68, 102, 104, 114, 165, 210, 242
Bliss Vocational Rehabilitation Center,
102, 243
Bliss Workshop, 176
Board of Visitors, 163, 189, 191, 195
boardinghouses, 176
Bogh, Richard, 243
Booth, William R., 195–196, 204
Boulos Property Management, 232
Boutilier, Mickey, 186, 197, 198, 199
Bowman, Peter W., 6, 121, 242
    appointment of, 79, 85–86
    budget under, 90, 103–104, 109
    on care for severely retarded, 112–117
    commendation of, 176
    controversies surrounding, 117–119
    discharges under, 96–97
    employees and, 87–88, 89, 90–91, 133
    expectations of, 86–87
    impact of, 238
    medical care under, 92–96
    new buildings and, 101–102
    population under, 87, 98, 101
    programs under, 101–102
    on sterilization, 118
Boy Scouts, 41, 63, 69, 74p, 75
Brennan, Joseph E., 149
Brewster, Ralph O., 42
"A Brief History of Pineland Center"
    (Hoffman), xix
Brockway, Alta (Haskell), 16
Brunelle, Jim, 134
Bruns, Margaret, 147, 243
Buck, Pearl, 84, 145
budget
    after consent decree, 165
    under Bowman, 90, 103–104, 109
    community services and, 204
    under Vosburgh, 29, 49
Burchard A. Dunn School, 224–225
Bureau of Mental Retardation, 127, 197,
    199, 200, 211
    Pineland Center closing and, 205
Bureau of Public Lands, 138, 191

Burrow, Will, 154
buses, 107, 110, 169, 171

Caldwell, Bill, 115–116
Camp Tall Pines Foundation, 178. See also
    Tall Pines Day Camp
Campbell, Eddy Brophy, 181
Campbell, Spencer W., 87
Campfire Girls, 41, 63, 106
canine training program, 175
Caouette, Raymond, 123
Carey, Harris M., 40
Carpentry Building, 232
Carroll, Donnell P., 190–191, 200, 205, 212
Carroll (resident), 141
Carter, Gene, 199, 216
"A Case for Community Placement"
    (Hoffman), 98–100
cemetery, 107, 108, 188p, 228
Chafin, Darla, 206, 227
chapel, 102, 107, 170p, 174p, 183, 224,
    227–228, 232, 233p. See also All
    Faiths Chapel
charitable donations, 72
Charlie (resident), 42
Chase, Eleanor, 47–48
Children's Psychiatric Hospital, 92, 94, 97,
    98, 136, 138, 242, 243
Chitwood, Michael J., 209
chlorpromazine, 94, 95, 104
Christmas angels, 180–181, 182p
Christmas celebrations, 6p, 62, 63–64, 74,
    106, 111
Church, Olive, 89
Church World: Maine's Official Catholic
    Weekly, 125–130, 126p, 130
Clark, Lincoln, 167–168, 170, 243
class action suit, 144–148, 144–152,
    176–178, 243. See also consent
    decree
classrooms, 33p, 50p, 137p. See also school
    buildings
clocks, 37
clusters organization, 192
Cobb, William T., 4
Cohen, Richard S., 155

Cole, John N., 134
Collier's Brook, 15, 117
Collins, Joan, 204, 217
Commons Building, 172, 173
community-based facilities, 127, 151–152
community care, 169, 170, 200
community housing, 199, 201-202
Concannon, Kevin W., 130, 151, 154, 169,
        176, 186, 187, 215, 236, 243, 244
Conference Center, 171
Connor, Sam E., 62, 66–68
conscientious objectors, 64, 73
Consensus Panel, 205–206
consent decree, 159–171, 167–168, 184,
        197–199
    complaints with, 189–190
    response to abuse reports, 185–190
    treatment services under, 226–227
    See also class action suit
Consent Decree Panel, 189–190
Consumer Advisory Board, 162–163,
        185–186, 189, 197, 199
Cook, David, 150
Coombs, Harry S., 53
Cooper, Bill, 212
"Coping" (newsletter), 185–186
correspondence, 57, 71
Cote, Adrian A., 72
Court of Appeals for the First Circuit,
        U.S., 198–199. *See also* class action
        suit; consent decree
Crichton, Mary, 165, 200–201, 239
crime, 34, 35
    mental illness and, 61–62
    See also fires
Cromwell, Marion, 177
Cumberland Hall, 105, 136, 137–138,
        142p, 161, 172, 179, 242
Curtis, Kenneth, 139
Cushman, Archie, 47

dairy farm, 10, 15p
dances, 40
Davis, Bob, 191
Day Activity Center, 172
dayrooms, 29p

deaths, 71, 161, 186
degenerate colonies, 3, 21
Degerstrom, Ed (resident), 143
deinstitutionalization, 92, 97–100, 124,
        140–141, 166
    under consent decree, 162
    See also discharges; normalization
dentist, 38, 93
Department of Health and Welfare, 62,
        242
Department of Institutions, 62
Department of Mental Health, Mental
        Retardation and Substance Abuse
        Services, 226-227, 236
Department of Mental Health and
        Corrections, 118, 127, 135, 142,
        144, 162, 165, 243
Department of Mental Health and Mental
        Retardation, 165, 197, 214, 243
Deshaies, Roger, 197, 201, 202, 203, 204,
        211
destitute, 18, 20
developmentally disabled, 176. *See also*
        feeble-mindedness; mental retar-
        dation
dining hall, 8, 93p, 242, iip
direct care workers, 165–166, 196–197. *See*
        also attendants; employees;
        matrons
Dirigo House, 37, 50, 57, 213
disabilities
    terminology for, xviii
    See also developmentally disabled; fee-
        ble-mindedness; mental retar-
        dation
discharges, 19–20
    under Bowman, 96–97
    sterilizations and, 36, 48
    See also deinstitutionalization; normal-
        ization
discipline, 46–48, 76, 208
    of employees, 187–189, 237
    Ferri on, 189
District Court, U.S., 144–148, 152. *See also*
        class action suit; consent decree
domestic services, 70

Doris Anderson Hospital, 159
Doris Sidwell Hall, 102, 111, 242
dormitories, 2p, 7, 37, 49, 52p, 66–68, 82p
Douglas, Wayne, 218
Dow, Charles, 14
Doyle, Dorothy, 112
drama programs, 41, 63
driver education program, 101, 114p, 242
Duby, Lynn F., 227
duckhouse, 172
Dykinga, Jack, xvi

Education for all Handicapped Children
        Act (1975), 122
educational programs, 39, 40–42, 63–64,
        96, 101, 177–178
Edwards, William B., 45
Eisenhower, Dwight D., 94
electricity, 37, 84, 117
Elizarian, Harry, 243
employees
    advertisements for, 68
    under Bowman, 87–88, 89, 90–91, 133
    closing and, 206–207, 212–213,
        216–217, 219
    dances for, 40
    discipline of, 187–189, 237
    duties of, 28, 115–116
    Hichens committee and, 134
    housing for, 38–39, 65, 101–102
    interfacing and, 177
    population of, 87, 236
    reaction to complaints, 190
    turnover rate, 79
    under Vosburgh, 48–49
    wages of, 48, 100, 116
    See also attendants; direct care workers;
        matrons
Ernest (resident), 133
escapes, 19, 152
    under Kupelian, 68–70, 79
    under Vosburgh, 31–32, 44–48
Estabrook, Richard, 209, 226–227
eugenics, 24, 35, 56. See also sterilization
Evans, Dale, 84, 85
Fabian (singer), 102

Fairweather, Charles E., 177
family care homes, 176
farming, 7, 39-40, 84, 96, 138
    during World War I, 23–24, 24p
    See also Hill Farm; Valley Farm
Federation Village, 101, 105, 171, 232, 242
feeble-mindedness, 11
    heredity and, 15, 16, 34–36
    sterilization and, 24
    theories on prevention of, 60–61
    use of term, 43–44
    See also disabilities; mental retardation
Fellers, Ellie, xiv, 89, 102, 217, 218, 235,
        238
Fernald, Walter E., 3, 4, 34
Ferri, Joseph M., 130, 169, 178, 186–187,
        217, 243
    on Behavior Stabilization Unit, 188
    on discipline, 189
Fire Station, 232, 243
fires, 31–34
    and fire prevention, 60
    under Kupelian, 60, 68–70, 79
First International Conference on Mental
        Retardation (1959), xv, 94
fishpond, 96
Five Towns Post, 83
Flahive, William, 163
Ford, Edward, 104
Ford, Gerald R., 150
formal training, 30
Fortier, Cheryl E., 163
Foster, Clifton E., 232
Foster Grandparents, 184–185
Fourth of July celebrations, 63, 77, 125,
        180, 193, 215
Frank D. Self Foundation, Inc., 95, 180
Fred (resident), 181
Freeport Towne Square, 176–177, 181,
        205, 219p, 243

Gallant, Elaine, 161, 165–166, 180, 189,
        196–197, 207, 210, 219
Gamache, Jean, 69
gambling, 55
Gardiner, William Tudor, 43

Gartner, Victor, 166
Gelinas, Pauline T., 204–205
Gignoux, Edward T., 149, 151, 152, 155, 167, 168, 169, 170, 197–198
Giguere, Frederick, 210–211, 211p, 220
Gilliam, Eric, 216, 244
Girls Home, 16
Glover, Robert, 197, 200–201
Graham, Ned, 185
Gray, 5, 224
Gray Hall, 7, 136–137, 242
Great Depression, 49
Greenlaw, Norman U., 75, 78
Greenleaf, Harrison C., 62, 68
Gregory, David D., 152, 154–155, 167, 243
ground observation post, 83
group homes, 176, 208–209
Grover, Commissioner, 205–206
gymnasium, 102, 105, 243. *See also* Soucy Gymnasium

Haile, Diane, 206
Haney, Walter, 45
Hannaford Brothers, 181
Hanscom, Dr., 50
Hansen, Donald C., 140
Hartley, Donald L., 197, 203, 208, 214, 244
Haskell, Wayne, 97, 138, 183, 187, 190, 197
Hawkes, Dennis, 210–211
Hawkes, Sharon, 210
Hayden Infirmary, 94, 116
Hebert, Arthur A., 59
Hedin, Carl J., 242
    appointment of, 15
    attendants under, 18
    heredity and feeble-mindedness, 15, 16
    medical facilities under, 38
    trustees and, 18
Hedin Hospital, 38, 54, 93, 171, 236, 242
heredity, 15, 16, 24, 34
Herman, Mary J., 218
Hichens, Walter, 134, 135, 171
Hildreth, Horace A., 73
Hill, George, 9
Hill Farm, 2p, 6, 10, 16, 84, 96, 117, 242
Hillcrest Poultry Company, 101

"History of Pineland" (Kleinberg), xix
Hobbs, Mrs. Charles M., 72
Hoffman, John L., xix, 9, 19–20, 31, 98–100, 111, 128, 133, 141, 143, 149, 153, 155, 185
Holmes, Oliver Wendell, 35
homelife cottage, 102
Hood, Perry A., xix
Hornby, D. Brock, 198
Hospital Improvement Program, 128–129, 134
Hough, Howard O., 77
Huber, David G., 165
Hughes, Curtis, 44
Human Resources Committee, 204, 215
Human Rights Committee, 186, 188
hydrotherapy, 120p
hygiene, 30

ice-cutting, 26p, 83
industrial arts, 17, 39, 40, 61p
infirmary, 94, 128, 224–225
informal training, 30
inmates. *See* residents
insanity. *See* disabilities; feeble-mindedness; mental retardation
Intel Corporation, 229
interfacing, 177
intermediate care facilities, 176
Intermediate Care-Mentally Retarded (ICF/MR) units, 162
Inventing the Feeble Mind: A History of Mental Retardation in the United States (Trent), xvi, 85, 122, 123, 162

Jacobs, Charles, 223, 225
Johnny (resident), 42
Johnson, Frank M., 145–146
Joint Commission on Accreditation of Hospitals, 95, 149, 170, 186
Juvenile Defective Deficiency Act (1941), 73
juvenile delinquents, 72, 73

Kamber, Hannah, 114–115

Karwowski, Pinky, 160–161, 190
Kearns, William F., Jr., 118–119, 135, 139,
    140, 142
Kelsey, Walter L., 8
Kennedy Foundation, 104, 150
Kerry, John, 125–130
Kimball, Laurie, 209
King, Angus S., Jr., xi-xii, 223, 224, 225,
    227, 232
Kinnelly, Charlene, 154, 243
kitchen, 22, 40p, 242
Kleinberg, Judith, xix
Kupelian, Nessib S., 43, 44, 50, 242
    background of, 54–55
    death of, 79
    description of school, 59–61
    escapes and, 68–70, 79
    fires and, 60, 68–70, 79
    growth under, 56, 65–68, 84
    on Hitler, 60
    investigations under, 57-58, 73–78
    on marriage, 61
    population under, 76, 79
    programs under, 63–64
    retirement of, 79
    sterilization and, 56, 61
Kupelian, Phillip N., 57, 83–84
Kupelian Hall, 68, 78p, 89, 97p, 102, 104,
    112–117, 124, 131, 169, 189, 242,
    243

labor unions, 90–91, 125, 135–136,
    140–141, 143, 145, 150
landfill, 136
laundry, 37, 49, 99, 102, 242
Lausier, Annette, 210
Lausier, Conrad P., 131–133, 152
Lausier, Suzanne, 178
Leadbetter, George W., 43, 58, 61–62
learning disabilities, 122. See also feeble-
    mindedness; mental retardation
Lee, Jeffrey R., 148, 167, 192-193, 200, 239,
    244
Letchworth Village, 23
Levinson Center, 127, 129
Lewiston-Auburn Kiwanis Club, 144

Lewiston-Auburn Rotary Club, 118
Libby, Eleanor M. Chase, 47–48
Libby, Harry E., 47
Libby, Steve, 231
Liberty Group, 225
Libra Foundation, xiii, 229–234, 235, 244
library, 173–174
Little, Charles S., 23
Longley, James B., 139, 149, 186
Longley Center, 173, 232
Loveitt, Hazel, 116
Lowe, Christopher, 41

Macgowan, Carroll M. "Skip," 145, 147,
    164–165, 200, 237
Maine
    Bureau of Finance and Administrative
        Services, 223
    Bureau of Mental Retardation, 127,
        197, 199, 200, 205, 211
    Bureau of Public Lands, 138, 191
    Department of Health and Welfare, 62,
        242
    Department of Institutions, 62
    Department of Mental Health, Mental
        Retardation and Substance
        Abuse Services, 226–227, 236
    Department of Mental Health and
        Corrections, 118, 127, 135,
        142, 144, 162, 165
    Department of Mental Health and
        Mental Retardation, 165, 197,
        214
    government, 43, 118–119
    Health and Institutional Services
        Committee, 135
    mental retardation statistics, 187
Maine Advocacy Service, 214
Maine Association for Retarded Citizens,
    145
Maine Central Railroad, 69
Maine Federation of Women's Clubs,
    73–74, 105, 242
Maine Medical Association, 29, 30
Maine Olmstead Alliance for Parks and
    Landscapes, 224

Maine Rowdy Running Team, 181–182
Maine School for Feeble-Minded, 2p, 228,
    231, 242
    admittance to, 18–20
    Bliss and, 4-15
    early scandals at, 13-15
    establishment of, 4–7
    farming at, 7
    Hedin and, 15-24
    name change of, 37
    newspaper accounts of, 7–9, 10–13,
        16–17
    population of, 7, 9
    during World War I, 22–24
    See also Pineland Center; Pineland
        Hospital and Training Center;
        Pownal State School
"Maine School for Feeble-Minded,
    Pownal State School" (Sedgley),
    xix
Maine State Archives, 227
Maine State Committee on the Arts and
    Humanities, 179–180
Maine State Federated Labor Council, 109
Maine State Police, 175
Maintenance Building, 243
"Making the Best of It" (film), 39, 45
Malaga Island, 3, 20–22, 228
Malthy, Sharon, 179
Manning, Peter, 197
manual training, 39, 50p
Margaret (resident), 218
marriages, 17, 40, 61
Marriner, Anna B., 40
Martti A. Wuori Workshop, 177
Massachusetts School for the Feeble-
    Minded, 4, 34
matrons, 28. See also attendants; direct
    care workers; employees
Matthews, Don, 215–216
Matthews, Sharon, 216
Mavis (resident), 153
Maynard, Thomas L., 119
McKernan, John, 191, 195, 204, 213
Medicaid, 170, 205
    community residence programs and,

201–202
medical care, 54, 71
    under Bowman, 92–96
    shortages in, 64
Medicare, 199
Memorial Craftsmen of Maine, 107, 108
Mental Health Law Project, 151
Mental Hospital Visitation Committee, 75
mental retardation
    attitudes toward, 3, 84–85, 121–125
    changing terminology of, 122–124
    classifications of, 11
    definition of, 122
    education, 96
    establishing institutions for, 3–4
    severe, 112–117
    statistics, 187, 199
    treatment services, 96, 226–227
    See also developmentally disabled; dis-
        abilities; feeble-mindedness
Mental Retardation Facilities and
        Community Health Centers
        Construction Act (1963), 104, 121
Michaud, Marcel, 124
mock trial, 44
modernization efforts, 43–44
Monroe, H. Jay, 110, 125, 129, 134, 226,
        239, 243
Moore, Louis F., 102, 109–112
Moore, Spencer, 173, 244
Morin, Marcel, 107
Morrison, Kenneth H., 113–114
Morse House, 16, 57
Morse Road, 225
mortuary, 38
motto, 28
movies, 43
Murnik, Linda, 224
music, 40, 41, 63
Muskie, Edmund S., 91, 94
Muskie Treatment Building, 102, 243
"My Special Boy" (poem), 167
Myerson, Abraham, 34

National Association for Retarded
    Children, 85

National Committee on Arts for the
Handicapped, 179
National Conference of Charities and
Correction, 4
National Institute of Mental Health, 104
Naval Reserves, U.S., 150
neglect, charges of, 57–58, 75–78, 186. *See
also* abuse, allegations of
Nemitz, Bill, 216
Nevin, Elizabeth H., 109
New England Basketball Tournament for
the Mentally Retarded, 123
New Gloucester, xviii, 5, 37, 212–213, 224
New Gloucester Cemetery Association,
228
New Gloucester Hall, 22, 52*p*, 172, 175,
242
New Gloucester Historical Society, xviii,
xx, 227
New Hampshire State Hospital, 95
Niedorf, Saul, 129–130, 136, 138
No Man's Land, 21
nonresidential programs, 176
normalization, 123–124, 134, 151–152,
162. *See also* deinstitutionaliza-
tion; discharges
North Yarmouth, xviii, 5
North Yarmouth Historical Society, 228
Norton, William, 180–181
Nottage, Mrs., 91
Noyce, Elizabeth, 231, 232
Nurses Home, 16, 49, 242
nursing homes, 176

Observer, 103*p*, 106*p*, 109, 111, 120*p*, 156*p*,
178–180, 198*p*, 236
October Corporation, 232
Olmstead, Fredrick Law, 224
Olmstead Brothers, 37–38
orphans, 18
outings, 131

Page, Harry O., 59
Pappanikou, Agisilaos J., 86, 101, 103, 117
parents, 90, 156, 161, 167–168, 169
Pineland Center closing and, 204–205,

206, 214, 216–217
See also Pineland Parents and Friends;
Pownal Parents and Friends
Parker, Carl Rust, 37–38
Parker, Susan, 197
Parsons, Julie, 240–241
patients. *See* residents
patients' rights, 146, 151–152
Payne, Frederick G., 74, 75, 119
pediatrics room, 193*p*
Peet, Melodie, 214, 215, 216
Perry D. Hayden Infirmary, 94
Perry Hayden Hall, 178, 224–225, 243
Peterson, Paul, 213, 214, 228, 244
Petit, Michael R., 155
pharmacy, 38
pheasants, 96
Phippsburg, 21
physical plant, 37–38
changes under Kupelian, 84
closing of, 212–213
potential uses for, 223–226, 229–234
under Zitnay, 171–175
physical training, 39, 40
Pine Tree Legal Assistance, 145, 146–148
Pineland: A Comprehensive Center for the
Developmentally Disabled, 159
Pineland Center, 222*p*, 225*p*, 243
administrative changes, 141–141
class action suit and, 144–156, 176-
178, 243
closing of, 195–219, 203*p*
early studies of, xix
location of, xviii
master key, 214*p*, 218
mementos of, 227–228
name change, xvii, 159
name of, 138
potential uses for, 223–226, 229–234
program guide, 161
records of, 227
resident population in 1990s, 205, 215
See also Maine School for the Feeble
Minded; Pineland Hospital
and Training Center; Pownal
State School

Pineland Chargers, 123
Pineland Closure Committee, 217–219
Pineland Conversion Committee, 223,
      225, 227–228, 230
Pineland Hospital and Training Center,
      94, 242
    investigations of, 112–117, 125–130,
        126*p*
    name change, 138
    name of, 87*p*
    philosophy of, 98
    professional training at, 102–103, 134
    statistics of, 117
    See also Maine School for the Feeble
        Minded; Pineland Hospital
        and Training Center; Pownal
        State School
Pineland Parents and Friends, 95, 107,
      112, 124, 150, 160–161, 171, 175,
      204, 206, 227, 228
Pineland Pops, 112
Pineland Program Standards, 151–152
"Pineland's 60 Years" (Hood), xix
Pioneers, 75
Plaisted, Frederick, 21
Platz Associates, 225
Pleury (resident), 32
Pollister, Arabella, 4
Pops Concert, 110
population, 236
    after legal settlement, 151
    under Bowman, 87, 98, 101
    deinstitutionalization and, 140
    of destitute, 18
    employee, 87, 236
    under Kupelian, 59, 65, 66, 68, 76, 79
    of Maine School for Feeble-Minded, 7,
        9, 18
    of orphans, 18
    postwar, 71–74
    in 1900s, 16
    in 1930s, 44, 49
    in 1940s, 56
    in 1980s, 162, 190, 199
    in 1990s, 205, 215
    under Vosburgh, 27, 30

    under Zitnay, 173
Porter, Ernestine, 76
Portland, 213–214
Portland Symphony Orchestra, 112
powerhouse, 37
Pownal, 5, xviii
Pownal Hall, 36*p*, 37, 38, 102, 104, 106,
      175, 242, 243
Pownal Parents and Friends, 90, 105
Pownal State School, 28, 70*p*, 242, xviii
    admittance to, 72–73
    investigations of, 73–78
    location of, 37
    name change, 94
    purpose of, 73
    See also Maine School for the Feeble
        Minded; Pineland Center;
        Pineland Hospital and
        Training Center
prisons, 191
private foundations, 104
professional training, 102–103, 134, 178
programs, 10, 117, 123, 178-180
    after consent decree, 176–178
    under Bowman, 101–102
    educational, 39, 40–42, 63–64, 96, 101,
        177–178
    under Kupelian, 63–64
    under Vosburgh, 39–42
psychiatric treatment, 92, 93, 95–96, 129
public relations department, 109–112
public schools, 122
punishment. *See* discipline

Questor, 223–224, 225*p*

radios, 43, 54
Raymond, Ralph, 110
recreational programs, 10, 117, 123,
      178–180
reeducation programs, 104
regional centers, 191
relay race, 181–182
Reorganization Plan Clusters, 190
Resident Council, 163
residential care, 124

residents
    accounts of, 31, 32, 42, 58, 60, 88, 98,
        128, 133, 141, 143, 153, 181,
        192–193, 218, 229
    advocacy groups for, 125, 162–164
    Pineland Center closing and, 200–211,
        216-217
    terminology for, xviii, 84
    wages for, 70, 130, 176
respite care assistance, 205
Retired Senior Volunteer Program,
    180–181
Ricker, Rose P., 86, 87, 90, 122, 173–174,
    183
Rogers, Roy, 84
Rosser, John, 129, 139, 140
runaways. See escapes
Ruth Ann (resident), 216–217

Sanborn, Lauren M., 34
sawmill, 71
School Administrative District 15,
    224–225
school buildings, 39. See also classrooms
Scruggs, Roberta, 181, 224
Sebago House, 22, 232, 242
Sedgley, E., xix
segregation, 30, 31
Self, Frank D., 105, 180
Self, Grace, 180
Sewall, Sumner, 62
sewing activities, 17
sex education, 101, 134
Shailer House, 16, 20p
sheltered workshop, 176–177, 181, 243
Small, Leo, 115–116
Smith, Kline & French, 104
smoking, 87, 189
soapbox derby, 107
Socialization Program, 111
Solomon, Harry, 92
Soucy, Walter J., 105–106, 107p
Soucy Gymnasium, 105, 130, 175, 243
special education classes, 122
Special Olympics, 121, 134, 179, 180, 212,
    243

speech and hearing labs, 104
Spiers, Alexander, 34
sports, 10
Spring Hobby and Handicraft Exposition,
    40
St. Gregory's Catholic Church, 227–228
Staples, Lindley M., 3, 4, 5–6
Staples Hall, 7, 16, 139, 242
State School for Boys, 19
State School for Girls, 19
sterilization, 24, 30, 31, 34–36, 48, 56, 61,
    66, 118, 164–165
Strong, Wendell, 143
Sturgis, Matthew, 231
sub-normal, 43–44
Superintendents
    Bliss, 4–15, 242
    Bowman, 6, 79, 85–119, 121, 176, 238,
        242
    Burrow, 154
    Concannon, 130, 151, 154, 169, 176,
        186, 187, 215, 236, 243, 244
    Ferri, 130, 169, 178, 186–187, 188, 189,
        217, 243
    Hedin, 15–24, 38, 242
    housing for, 41, 55p, 57
    Kupelian, 43, 44, 50, 54–79, 84
    Monroe, 110, 125, 129, 134, 226, 239,
        243
    Moore, 173, 244
    Peterson, 213, 214, 228, 244
    Vosburgh, 24, 27–50, 242
    Wurtz, 136–140, 144-148, 161, 243
    Zitnay, 151, 155, 161, 162, 166, 171-
        175, 243
supervised apartment programs, 176
support groups, 162–164
swimming pool, 109, 150, 150p, 243

Tall Pines Day Camp, 103p, 106, 112,
    132p, 134, 144, 178, 180, 212, 243
Tapley, Lance, 185–186
Task Force on Pineland Center Reuse, 223,
    244
Taylor, Henry (pseudonym), 31
therapeutic pool, 175

Thomas, Nancy L., 163, 201, 211, 237
"Those Who Knew" (Parsons), 240–241
Tierney, James, 186
tobacco, 31
tranquilizers, 94, 95
treatment, 96, 193
    under consent decree, 226–227
    under Vosburgh, 30
Tremblay, Mary Beth, 200, 206, 208–209, 233
Trent, James W., Jr., xvi, 85, 122–123, 162
True, Betty, 87
Trustees, 18, 19, 43
Tyson, Forrest C., 34

unitization, 138–139, 140
University of Maine, 178

Valley Farm, 10, 12p, 16, 96, 117, 146p, 243
vans, 107, 171
Very Special Arts Festival, 179
Vocational Building, 242
vocational education, 96, 242
Volunteer Institute and Awards Program, 106
volunteers, 105–109, 107p, 110, 112, 130, 133–134, 144, 180–185
Vosburgh, Beulah M., 33
Vosburgh, Stephen E., 242
    appointment of, 24
    budget under, 49
    death of, 50
    disciplinary measures under, 46–48
    employees under, 48–49
    escapes under, 31-32, 44–48
    family of, 33
    fires and, 31–34
    growth under, 37-39, 49
    name of school and, 37
    population under, 27, 30
    praise for, 27, 28
    programs under, 39–42
    on sterilization, 35–36
Vosburgh Hall, 171, 175, 242

W., Harry (resident), 88
Wahl, Mabel and Mildred, 48
Walker, Richard and Theresa, 128
Walter E. Fernald State School, 6
Waltz, Lee, 108
Ware, Shirley (resident), 218
Welch, Ronald, 197, 203
Wells, Owen W., xiii, 224, 229–234
Westbrook Jaycees, 107
Weston, Mrs. C.A., 4
wheelchairs, 110
White, Sonya, 216
Whitney, Pennie, 169
Wilcox, Nancy L., 129, 133, 149, 177, 183
Witham, Edward P., 242
Witham Pond, 172, 179, 194p, 217
Wolfensberger, Wolf, 123
Woodfords Club, 30
Woodruff, Neville, 146, 148–149, 151, 152, 154, 168–169, 195, 206, 217
woodworking shop, 172
Work Activities Program, 115, 176
work training program, 101
World War I, 22–24
World War II, 53, 63–65
    postwar difficulties, 71–74
Wuori, Martti, 146, 152, 158p
Wurtz, Betty, 184
Wurtz, Conrad R., 243
    administrative changes under, 142
    appointment of, 136
    deinstitutionalization and, 140, 141
    programs under, 161
    survey of buildings, 136–138
    unitization plan, 138–139, 140
    U.S. District Court and, 144–148
Wyman, Charles L., 186, 191, 192–193
Wyman, Charles O., 20, 33p, 39, 45–46, 69, 70, 192–193, 218, 218p, 229, 234

X-rays, 87

Yarmouth Hall, 37, 76, 147, 227, 230p, 242

Zitnay, George A., 151, 155, 243
    on consent decree, 161, 166
    on deinstitutionalization, 162
    plant improvements, 171–175
    population under, 173

About the Author

Richard S. Kimball is a freelance writer and photographer who lives on Morse Road in New Gloucester, Maine, just two miles from Pineland Center. A native of Orono, he graduated from high school there in 1958. He received a bachelor's degree in history from Harvard College in 1962 and a master's degree in journalism from Columbia University in 1968.

Between college and graduate school, Kimball was an officer in the United States Air Force. Later he worked as a reporter, columnist, and editor with the Portland, Maine, newspapers; and as a writer, acquisitions editor, and editor in chief for J. Weston Walch, Publisher, a Portland-based producer of supplementary educational materials distributed throughout the United States and Canada. In 1995 he and his wife, Tirrell, formed Kimball Associates, a firm offering a wide range of editorial services.

Kimball's recent freelance writing credits include a series of reproducible life-skills books for adults and youth with low reading skills, various middle school curricula, an exploration of creativity, and an adult human sexuality curriculum.